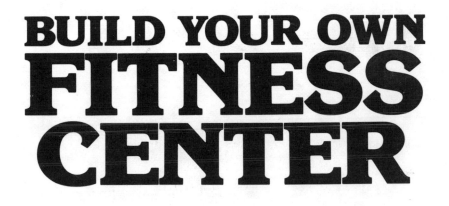

BUILD YOUR OWN FITNESS CENTER

No. 1828
$18.95

BUILD YOUR OWN
FITNESS CENTER

DAN RAMSEY

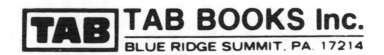

TAB BOOKS Inc.
BLUE RIDGE SUMMIT, PA. 17214

Other TAB Books by the Author

No. 1263 *How To Be A Disc Jockey*
No. 1458 *Building a Log Home from Scratch or Kit*
No. 1508 *The Complete Book of Fences*
No. 1568 *How to Forecast Weather*
No. 1578 *Doors, Windows and Skylights*
No. 1598 *Kerosene Heaters*
No. 1658 *How to Forecast Weather*
No. 2339 *Student Pilot's Solo Practice Guide*

FIRST EDITION

FIRST PRINTING

Copyright © 1985 by TAB BOOKS Inc.

Printed in the United States of America

Library of Congress Cataloging in Publication Data

Ramsey, Dan, 1945—
Build your own fitness center.

Includes index.
1. Sports facilities—Design and construction.
I. Title.
GV401.R35   1984   690'.58043   84-16429
ISBN 0-8306-0828-1
ISBN 0-8306-1828-7 (pbk.)

Contents

This book is dedicated to Byron, with special love.

Acknowledgments

Many people contributed to the completeness of this book including: Sunbeam Leisure Products Co.; Georgia-Pacific Corp.; AMF American, MacLevy Products Corp.; Exercycle Corp.; National Spa and Pool Institute; Western Wood Products Association; American Plywood Association; The President's Council on Physical Fitness; Departments of the Army, Navy, and Air Force; U.S. Department of Agriculture; The Fitness Shop of Portland, Oregon; and especially Rick Pathman for his artistic contribution.

Introduction

Fitness is a multibillion-dollar-a-year business. Fitness centers, health spas, and gymnasiums are sprouting up across the country to satisfy the public's desire to "stay in shape."

As a do-it-yourselfer, you can enjoy twice the exercise by building and using your own private fitness center. *Build Your Own Fitness Center* offers simple, step-by-step instructions and plans for an exercise room, weight room, gym equipment, indoor courts, sauna, fitness bath, and outdoor fitness center. You'll also learn how to choose and use tools, how to add a room, soundproof, panel, and paint. And you'll learn how to use your fitness center, with tips on exercise and physical conditioning. Plus, there are more than 70 sources and resources in the Appendices.

1

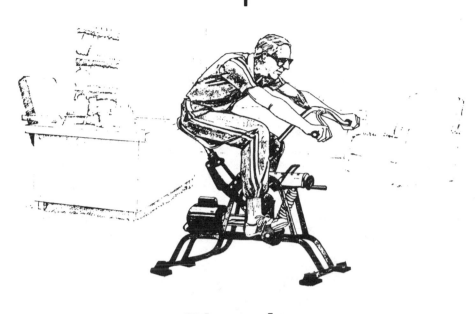

Planning

PHYSICAL FITNESS MEANS MORE THAN having strong muscles and great endurance. It means enjoying the best possible health plus the capacity to perform everyday tasks effectively and to meet emergencies as they arise. It is all relative, because handicapped people may be physically fit within the limitations imposed by their handicaps. Your goal should be to reach and maintain a level of physical fitness that is maximal for you.

Physical fitness has two basic aspects: *medical fitness*, which means having a sound, healthy body; and *dynamic fitness*, which is your capacity for action. The first is determined by a medical examination and the second by tests of physical performance.

You can have one aspect of physical fitness without the other. For example, suppose you get a "clean bill of health" from your physician, but you can't stand even slight exertion without distress. In this case you may be healthy, but you aren't physically fit because you lack the capacity for action. On the other hand, you may be an athlete who performs well but has an undetected health problem. If so, you aren't physically fit because you are not healthy. For this reason your action capacity, although good, may be below your potential.

While dynamic fitness is important to your health, you should first make sure you are medically fit before beginning your fitness program. If you haven't had one recently, get a medical checkup and set up a program for regular medical care. Watch your diet too. Proper nutrition is vital in achieving and maintaining physical fitness. If you are dieting, make sure you are getting a balanced diet. Medical fitness also requires rest. Rest is important in maintaining physical fitness because continuous activity at a high level produces fatigue and chronic strain if there is no respite. Relaxation in a quiet place or a change of activity is restful and should supplement a sufficient amount of sleep daily.

YOUR PERSONAL FITNESS CENTER

While most adults agree that physical fitness is important to an abundant life, we often put off a regular exercise program because we don't have a regular place and time in which to do it. It's often true that if we had a fitness center of our own—ranging from a corner of the bedroom to a complete gymnasium room or outdoor courts—we would find the time to utilize it.

The decision to plan and install a personal fitness center is a good one. First, it involves a commitment to better health. Following through on a decision to set aside space for dynamic fitness will give you the motivation to set aside the time for a regular fitness session.

Second, installing your own fitness center offers an enjoyable group of exercises: assembling parts, cutting and nailing, bolting, lifting, pulling. You'll especially get a workout if you decide to remodel a basement or add a room to your home for your personal fitness center (Fig. 1-1).

Third, your completed fitness center can be a source of pride. Just as you planned and implemented your fitness center, you can be confident of planning and implementing a successful fitness program.

Best of all, planning and installing your

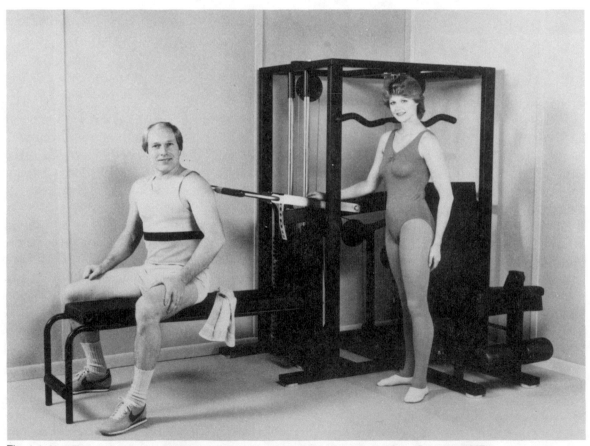

Fig. 1-1. Installing and using your personal fitness center can be both easy and fun. (Courtesy AMF)

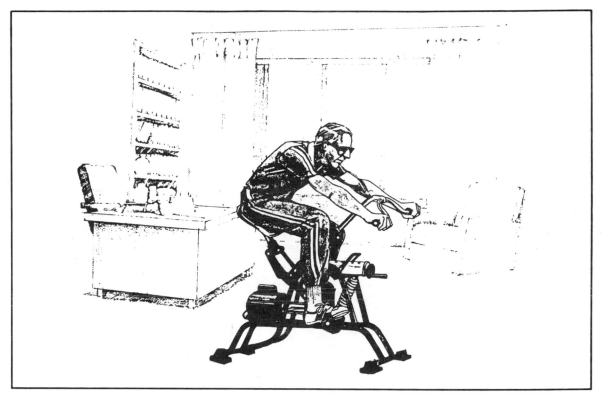

Fig. 1-2. A piece of fitness equipment set up in your home or office can be the beginning of your fitness center. (Courtesy Exercycle)

personal fitness center, large or small, offers you, your family, and your friends an enjoyable way to put pleasure into what may often seem like a lot of work (Fig. 1-2).

THE IMPORTANCE OF DYNAMIC FITNESS

Although physical fitness depends on medical fitness, this book will emphasize the dynamic fitness achieved through regular vigorous exercise at your personal fitness center. Americans today are healthier in many ways than their ancestors, but their lifestyle provides them with much less exercise. Many advances of modern technology—from electric can openers to power steering in automobiles—have made life easier and more comfortable but much less physically demanding. Why worry about strength and en-

durance in a push-button age? Because in order to keep healthy, your body needs the physical activity you miss when labor-saving devices do all the work.

When the physical demands of daily living are minimal, you need to seek opportunities to exercise for many reasons. The strength and endurance developed through regular vigorous exercise enable you to perform daily physical tasks with relative ease. Routine activity doesn't allow you to increase your capacity to work or to develop any physical reserve capacity. Agility and skill gained through the practice of varied movements can help you achieve an economy of movement that lessens the physical effort required for routine tasks.

Inactivity is often as important as over-eating in creeping overweight. Physical activity not only helps to control your weight by burning up excess calories (Table 1-1), but aids in the prevention of such degenerative diseases as hardening of the arteries, diabetes, and arthritic—diseases that are common and serious in the obese (Fig. 1-3).

Table 1-1. Energy Expenditure by a 150-Pound Person in Various Activities.

ENERGY EXPENDITURE BY A 150 POUND PERSON IN VARIOUS ACTIVITIES *	
Activity	*Gross Energy Cost-Cal per hr.*
A. Rest and Light Activity..**50–200**	
Lying down or sleeping..	80
Sitting	100
Driving an automobile..	120
Standing	140
Domestic work	180
B. Moderate Activity **200–350**	
Bicycling (5½ mph)...	210
Walking (2½ mph)..	210
Gardening	220
Canoeing (2½ mph)..	230
Golf	250
Lawn mowing (power mower)......................................	250
Bowling	270
Lawn mowing (hand mower)..	270
Fencing	300
Rowboating (2½ mph)...	300
Swimming (¼ mph)...	300
Walking (3¾ mph)...	300
Badminton	350
Horseback riding (trotting)..	350
Square dancing	350
Volleyball	350
Roller skating	350
C. Vigorous Activity ....**over 350**	
Table tennis	360
Ditch digging (hand shovel)...	400
Ice skating (10 mph)...	400
Wood chopping or sawing..	400
Tennis	420
Water skiing	480
Hill climbing (100 ft. per hr.)......................................	490
Skiing (10 mph)...	600
Squash and handball...	600
Cycling (13 mph)...	660
Scull rowing (race)..	840
Running (10 mph)..	900

The standards represent a compromise between those proposed by the British Medical Association (1950), Christensen (1953) and Wells, Balke, and Van Fossan (1956). Where available, actual measured values have been used; for other values a "best guess" was made.

Dynamic fitness can help to protect you in an emergency. Improved strength and physical endurance may help you to survive perilous situations. The development of quicker reaction time may enable you to avert a potentially serious accident.

Good posture and good muscle tone can help you to avoid the type of low-back strain associated with sedentary living. Enjoyable exercise provides relief from tension and is an antidote to irritation, frustration, and other pressures. If you're physically fit, you'll be able to relax more effectively. You will acquire poise and grace by learning to move efficiently. This will improve your appearance and help you feel more at ease in social situations. Feeling physically fit will improve your self-image.

HOW MUCH EXERCISE?

The answer to this question depends on the advice of your physician. It should be based on the results of your medical examination, your age, your physical condition, and your general reaction to physical activity. If you're out of physical condition, a safe rule is to start slowly with whatever exercise you undertake and increase the intensity and duration as your fitness improves. In time, you should be able to do with ease what was hard for you in the beginning.

Exercise periods need to be long enough and hard enough to tax your body to some extent. The body has built-in safety valves, and reasonable fatigue is not harmful. The ability to recuperate after physical activity is a good guide for determining how strenuously you should exercise. Breathlessness and pounding of the heart are natural reactions to exercise, but your pulse and rate of breathing should return to normal within a few minutes after you have stopped. Any feeling of weak-

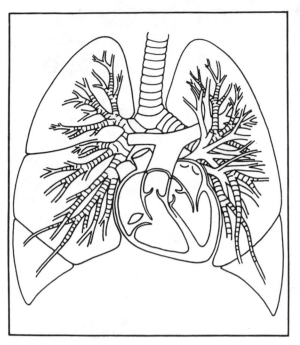

Fig. 1-3. The cardiovascular pulmonary system. (Courtesy Exercycle)

ness or fatigue should disappear within an hour or so. Exercise of appropriate intensity should not interfere with your sleep or leave you feeling unduly stiff the next day, except for the first few days after you start a new program.

Remember that exercising only once a week yields nothing but sore muscles. Pick activities that you can perform more regularly, three to five times a week. You don't have to do the same thing every time you exercise. Variety adds spice to your exercise schedule.

Some people aren't in a position to indulge in vigorous activities on a regular basis. If you're one of these people, try to look forward to a brisk daily walk supplemented by a series of brief exercises that can be done at your fitness center. First thing in the morning—before breakfast—is a time many people find convenient, since nothing else is scheduled and interruptions are few. Before long, you'll find that this period becomes as much a part of your daily routine as eating your meals and reading your newspaper.

WHAT KINDS OF EXERCISE?

The best forms of exercise for you will depend on your age, physical condition, physician's recommendations, and individual preference. Select activities that you already enjoy or think you might enjoy. Don't rule any out until you've given them a try. They should fit into your daily schedule and should be vigorous enough to give you the effect you need.

The type of fitness equipment you choose to build or install depends upon your personal physical fitness goals. You can plan and build a simple exercise room that offers space for aerobics or calisthenics with little or no equipment (Figs. 1-4 through 1-19). Or you may want to install a complete weight room. You may want to build up a room of gymnasium equipment that you've bought or built. Or maybe physical fitness to you means indoor Ping-Pong, racquetball, and other sports. Your fitness center can also include an indoor or outdoor sauna or a fitness bath complete with whirlpool, hot tub, or wet room. You can also

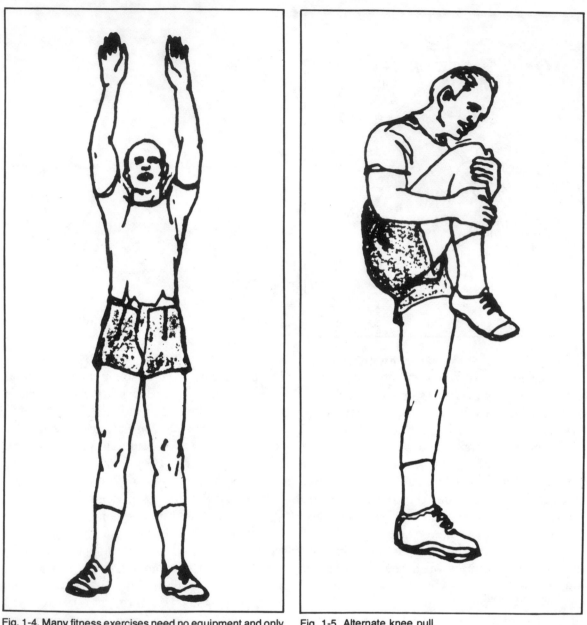

Fig. 1-4. Many fitness exercises need no equipment and only a small amount of floor space, such as the standing reach and bend.

Fig. 1-5. Alternate knee pull.

build your own outdoor fitness center including baseball, basketball, tennis, handball, and other sports courts. All these and many other exercise options will be offered in the coming pages of this book—complete with instructions on how to use common tools, how to remodel, and how to add on.

Your exercise program should be bal-

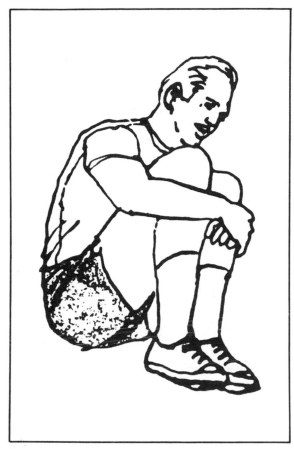

Fig. 1-6. Double knee pull.

anced, if possible. Part of the program, such as brisk walking, jogging, or swimming, should exercise your heart and lungs especially. Other parts should be directed toward improving strength, agility, flexibility, balance, timing, coordination, and muscle tone.

There are four main approaches to exercise, any or all of which you can use to reach your goal. First, exercise according to a regular schedule. Plan to go through a specific and individual exercise regimen each morning or every other day.

Second, step up your ordinary physical activities. Walk briskly. Move a little faster. Breathe deeper.

Third, find greater opportunities for physical activity. Climb the stairs rather than ride the elevator. Take a walk during your lunch hour.

Finally, supplement your daily activity with some form of physical recreation, such as a game of tennis. You may decide to take a weekly swimming class or build a simple handball court at home. Recognize your need and desire for enjoyable exercise and begin planning your own fitness center.

YOUR OWN FITNESS CENTER

Given enough knowledge, time, space, and money you could build the ultimate personal physical fitness center. It would have the latest in dynamic fitness and sports equipment,

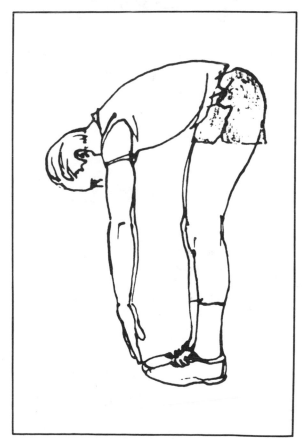

Fig. 1-7. Flexed-leg back stretch.

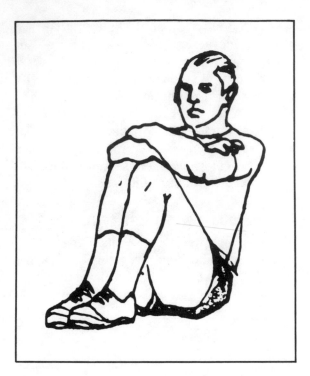

Fig. 1-8. Sit-up with arms crossed.

Fig. 1-9. Sit-up
with fingers laced.

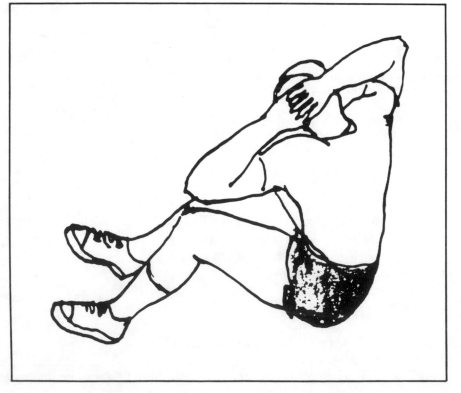

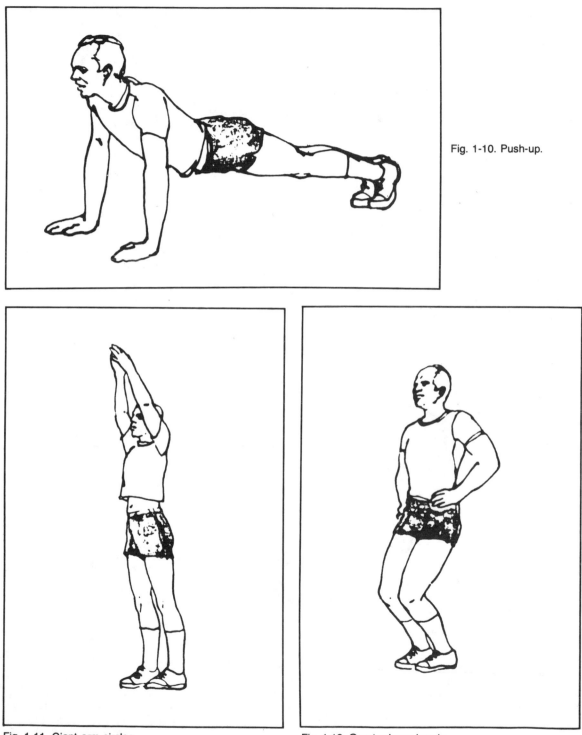

Fig. 1-10. Push-up.

Fig. 1-11. Giant arm circles.

Fig. 1-12. Quarter knee bends.

9

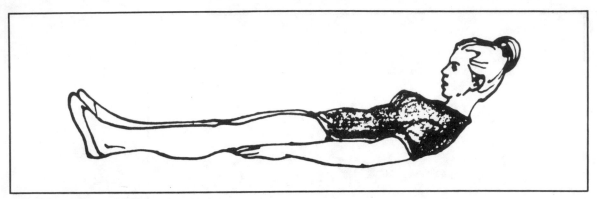

Fig. 1-13. Head and shoulder curl.

piped-in music, subtle lighting, and maybe an instructor or two.

Most of us are limited in at least one, and probably all, of these elements: knowledge, time, space, and money. So we do the best we can with what we have. Knowledge is increased through books and talking with fitness center owners and equipment dealers. Time is always a problem, but its limitations can be mastered to build a useful fitness center. Space can be used more efficiently or even increased. Money, normally in short supply, can be used more efficiently by understanding what you want and how best to get it. It's a matter of being a good consumer.

Maybe you feel like you don't know quite

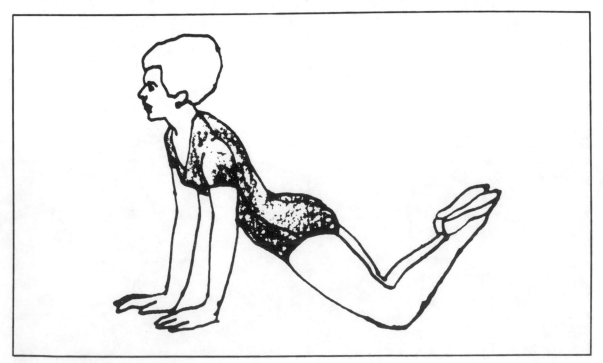

Fig. 1-14. Knee push-up.

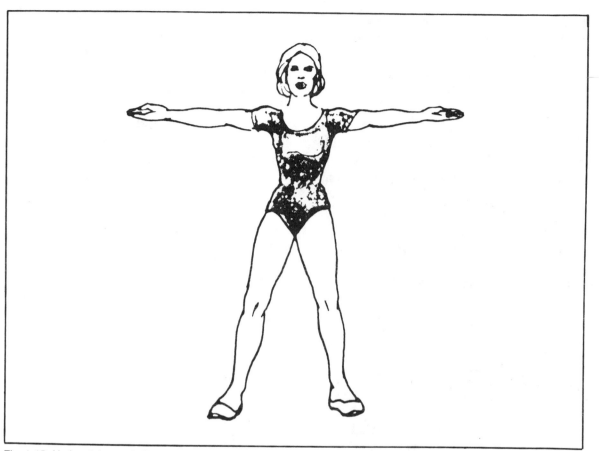

Fig. 1-15. Horizontal arm circles.

what you want or how to go about getting it. Considering the many options offered in this book should help solve that problem. Your physical condition and personal preferences will also dictate the best type of fitness center for your home or office. A realistic look at the elements may dictate that an exercise bicycle in the corner of your bedroom will be your complete fitness center. Calisthenics may completely turn you off. You may opt for a basketball half-court located in your driveway—or a volleyball court in your backyard. Take a closer look at the type of exercise you enjoy most as you plan your personal fitness center. Keep in mind, too, that others may be using the fitness center: spouse, children, relatives, and friends.

Maybe you feel you're just not a do-it-yourselfer; that you lack the skills to build a balance beam or remodel your basement. Then this book is especially written for you. The next chapter will outline the tools and techniques needed to build or install the projects suggested later in the book, plus show you how to make room in your home or office for them. A few basic tools are all that are needed to build most projects.

Planning your fitness center requires that you discover how much time you have for both building and using it. Autumn is often the best time to build an indoor fitness center that can be used through the winter. Spring is a good time to install outdoor saunas, hot tubs, and outdoor courts. But most of these projects can be built any time of the year in many areas of the country.

Consider your current schedule and your calendar for the amount of time you'll be able to devote to building your own fitness center. You may be able to offer four hours each Saturday morning, or an hour each evening, or maybe just a one-day block of time. The time available will help dictate whether you will be adding a room, remodeling, building your own equipment, or maybe just clearing away some furniture to make room for your rowing machine.

The space available within you home or office will also be important to planning your personal fitness center. If you live in a small urban apartment you may only have enough room to drag out the exercise bike from the closet. Or you may have a weight bench and weight rack in an extra bedroom. Maybe you have an unfinished basement or attic that offers potential space for a sauna. Or maybe you are pretty serious about this and have decided to add a fitness room to your home complete with equipment and bath. Permanence and portability are dictated by your life-style: renter, homeowner, condo resident.

How much can you spend? Your personal fitness center doesn't have to cost a dynamically-developed arm and a leg. It can be

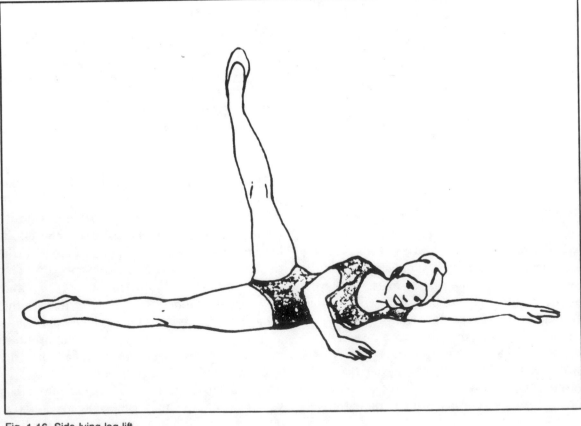

Fig. 1-16. Side-lying leg lift.

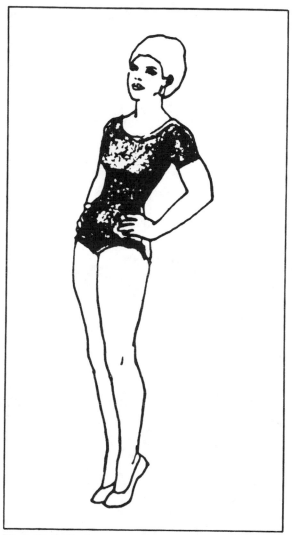

Fig. 1-17. Heal raises.

as inexpensive as a jump rope or exercise mat and as costly as a custom-designed gymnasium and bath. You may decide to start with nothing more than a remodeled basement, a weight bench, and a calorie chart, adding on to your fitness center as interests and cash dictate.

The first step then in building your own fitness center is planning it—and planning requires that you know what you want, how to get it, how much time you have to put it together and use it, how much space you have to install it, and how much money you have to spend on it. You may have some or all of the answers to these questions right now, or you may decide to read a whole book before even planning your fitness center. You will discover better, easier, and less costly ways of installing and using your personal fitness center as you continue reading.

FINDING ROOM

One of the greatest limitations on many fitness center planners is space. The time available and cash needed can often be modified to fit goals, but an 800-square foot apartment cannot. It's more a matter of budgeting space. Let's take a look at some of the possibilities for finding the space you need to install your fitness center.

The first thing to do is map out your current living space. Use a tape measure, pencil, and paper to draw a rough layout of your home or apartment. Refer to house blueprints if you have them. Draw the layout to scale such as 1 inch equals 2 or 4 feet. Be sure to include unfinished or unused living space: garage, attic, basement, half-basement, porch, deck. Mark the location of doors and windows so that you know how much usable wall space you have.

Don't be discouraged if it seems as if every inch of space is already in use. Rearranging rooms and furnishings can often free up space for an adequate fitness center. You may also decide to remodel or add on.

Before you consider talking with the lumber yard, take a closer look at your living space layout (Fig. 1-20). Can the functions of two rooms be combined into one (Fig. 1-21)? Can the family room and living room be combined to free up one or the other? Can excess furniture from one bedroom be moved to another to offer needed space (Fig. 1-22)? Is

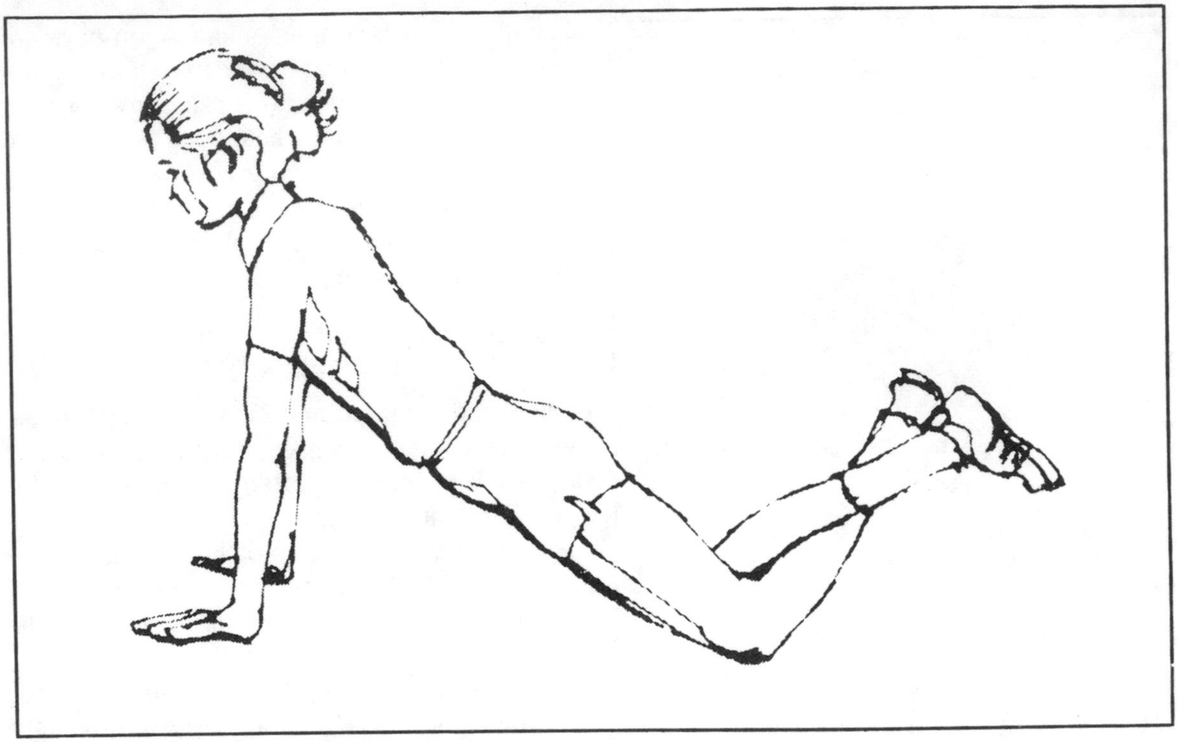

Fig. 1-18. Youngster fitness: knee push-up.

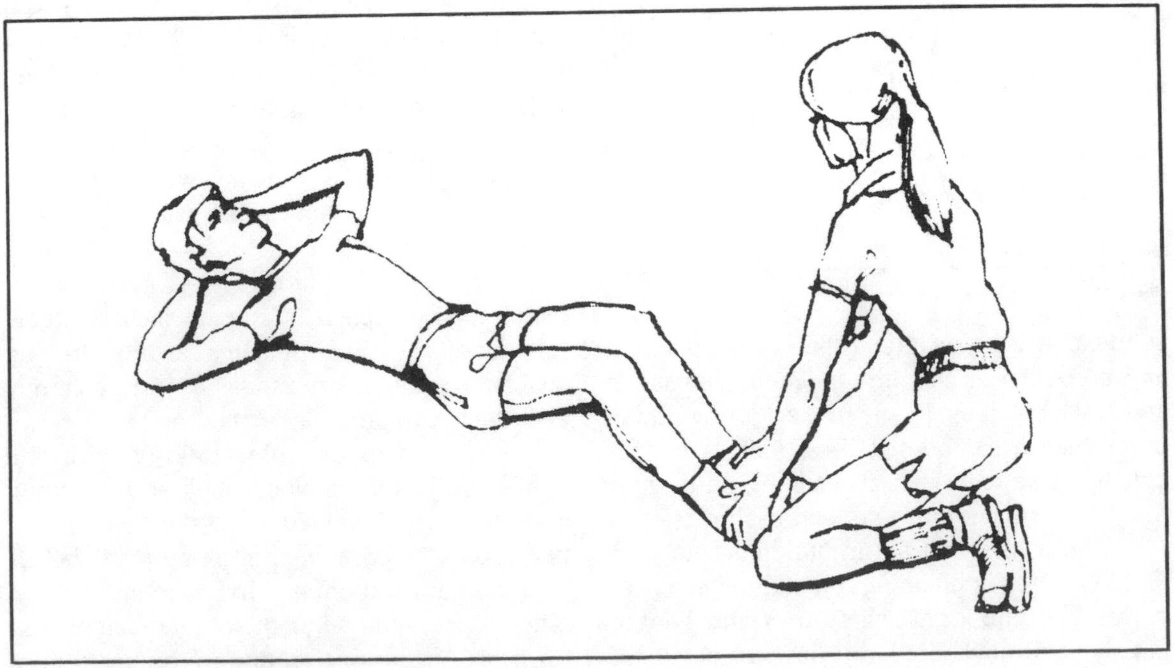

Fig. 1-19. Youngster fitness: assisted sit-up.

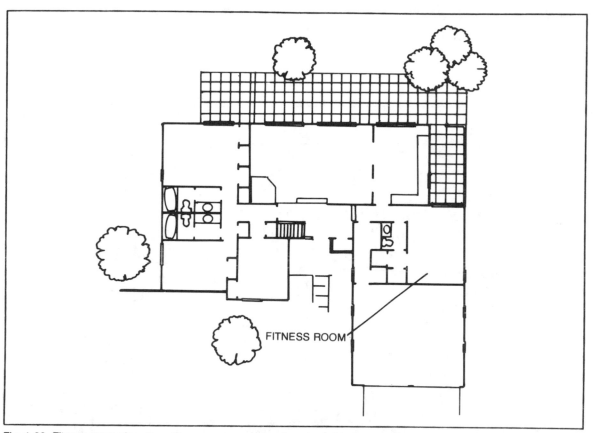

Fig. 1-20. Fitness room plan. Your fitness room can often be adapted into your current home layout.

the corner of the garage available for a small fitness center? Can you simply install shelving in a closet where fitness equipment can be stored between uses? Take a fresh look at your living quarters and ask others to offer suggestions. Sometimes a second opinion will offer the solution to your space problems.

USING THE BASEMENT

The most popular room for a personal or family fitness center is often the basement (Fig. 1-23) which can offer the greatest amount of unused, yet usable space. Everything you need for even the most developed fitness center is usually at hand: walls, floor, ceiling, wiring, plumbing, and heat.

Some homes include an unfinished basement with a cold cement slab floor and bare walls or even a dirt floor. Don't be discouraged. In coming chapters you'll learn how to seal up your basement, install new flooring and subflooring, insulate and panel walls, and even add heating, wiring, and plumbing if needed. Cabinets can also be installed to store equipment and games.

MOVING TO THE ATTIC

The second location to consider is the attic of your home. Many older homes include attics that were intended for storage but can be easily remodeled to become useful living space or a fitness center with a minimum of materials and effort. Some newer homes have smaller attics,

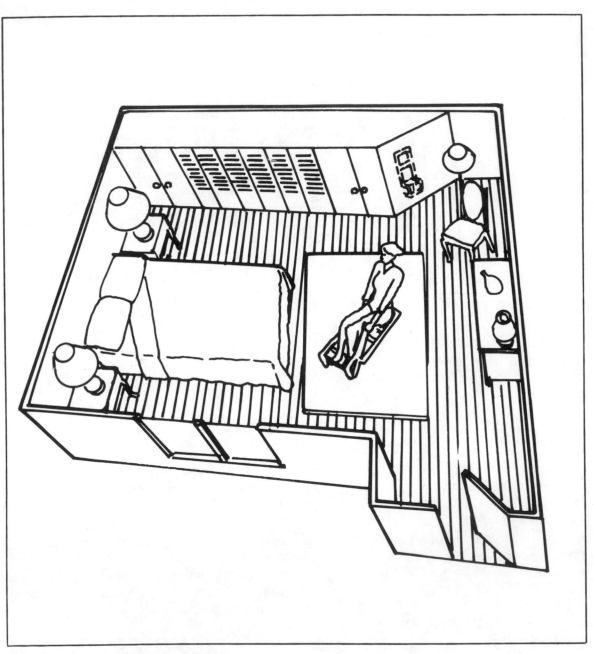

Fig. 1-21. Layout of a bedroom/fitness room.

but they too can be utilized indirectly. They can store the unused furnishings that will be replaced by your fitness equipment. A small attic may even have enough headroom for lim-ited use as a fitness center once a pull-down stairway is installed for access.

Another possibility considered by many fitness center builders is the addition of a

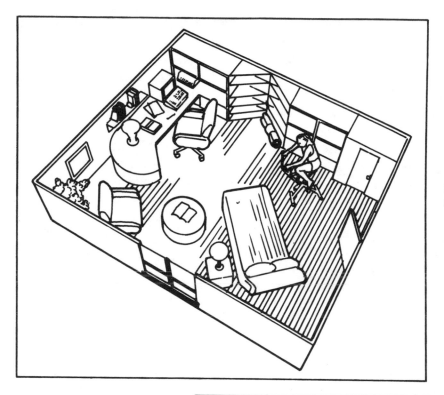

Fig. 1-22. Layout of
an office/fitness room.

Fig. 1-23. Layout of
a basement/fitness room.

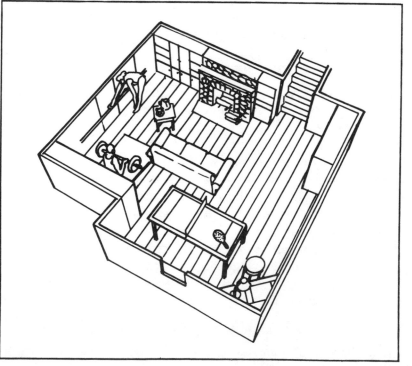

dormer to offer extra headroom. You'll find complete instructions on how to plan and install a dormer in your attic later in this book.

CONVERTING THE PORCH

Many porches offer the room needed for a fitness center with little modification. Some will only require a screen enclosure in milder climates. Others may need one or two walls added to enclose them for use. The necessary wiring and plumbing may be nearby, minimizing the need to bring utilities the longer distances that may be needed for a basement or attic installation. This modified porch can serve other purposes and help justify the costs. Your porch could become a greenhouse, a storage room, a hobby room, or even an extra bedroom.

If you're considering converting your porch into a fitness center, look carefully at the number and size of walls, windows, and utilities required for the remodeling job. It may be more economical than cleaning up the attic or using the basement—or it may not.

CONVERTING THE GARAGE

One effective way of gaining an inexpensive fitness center or recreation room at a moderate cost is by converting all or part of the garage, Again the walls, flooring, ceiling, and utilities are often available for a simple remodeling that can be done in a weekend. If your garage is large enough, you may decide to enclose a corner with a simple wall and throw down a rug for your fitness room. You may want to move the car(s) outside and remodel the entire garage into one or more living spaces for fitness, recreation, and storage. This too will be covered in greater detail later.

ADDING ON

Others have simply run out of space. There's no basement, attic, porch, or garage available for the luxury of a personal fitness center. In this case, many serious fitness buffs consider making an addition or extension to their home. This requires a great deal more planning, time, and money, but may be a bargain if the space can be utilized for other purposes. The addition could be an extra bedroom and fitness center. It could become a family room, hobby room, or sewing room depending on needs.

Adding on is more expensive than the conversion of an existing space, but it can usually be financed with a home improvement loan or second mortgage at lower interest rates than otherwise available. It can make a permanent and valuable improvement to the property.

The most popular sizes of additions are 16 by 16 feet and 12 by 20 feet, but smaller and larger add-ons can be planned depending on home layout. The best location to add on to your home is often at a bedroom, family room, or the end of a hallway. You can also move an existing room to the addition and make the old room your new fitness center. The possibilities are endless, but they begin with carefully reviewing your home layout.

SPACE REQUIREMENTS

How much space will you need for your fitness center? Space is like money: it seems that you always need more than you have. A good rule is to gain as much space as you can afford. If you're really serious about physical fitness, are involved in weight lifting, gymnastics, or sports, and know your requirements, you may decide to add a room or make a major investment in a room remodeling. But maybe this is your first shot at a regular exercise routine and you're not sure you have the interest or money for a complete fitness room. You can usually justify a modified fitness center or location

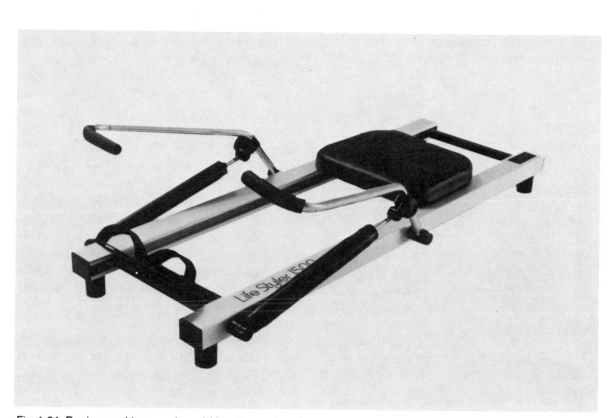

Fig. 1-24. Rowing machines can be quickly set up and easily stored out of the way. (Courtesy AMF)

within your home or apartment where fitness equipment can be used and stored.

If you haven't built or purchased your fitness equipment yet, but have an idea of what you want, you can visit a fitness or sports shop and measure the space needed by selected equipment on display. A salesperson can often be helpful in laying out the equipment space requirements and even a suggested clustering for greatest efficiency.

Rowing machines, weight benches, rebounders, and similar equipment (Figs. 1-24 through 1-27) usually only need a space of 3 by 6 feet each for setup. However, access room and accessory storage room is also needed. A 30-to-40-square-foot area should be allowed for each of these pieces of fitness equipment. This means that a fitness center with a weight bench, a rowing machine, and a jogging exer-

ciser should be from 90 to 120 square feet—9 by 10 feet to 10 by 12 feet. If necessary, these three pieces of fitness equipment could be squeezed into a smaller space, but they may require movement each time one is used. Your fitness center will be a compromise between the space needed and the space available.

Once you've selected the equipment you'll install or build you can draw them into your housing layout to see how they fit in (Figs. 1-28 through 1-31). You may want to cut out scaled replicas of the equipment and access space needed to lay out on the plan. Equipment can then be easily moved for the most efficient locations.

GETTING HELP

If your fitness center project is very large, you may decide to get help with the planning, re-

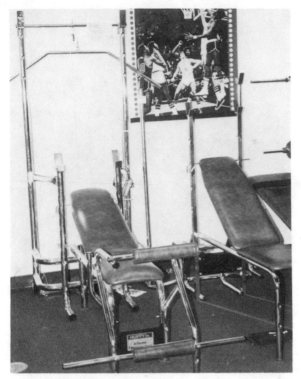

Fig. 1-25. Typical weight bench.

modeling, and installation of space and equipment. You may decide to have a contractor implement your addition, or you might want to do your own contracting and hire the subcontractors. All are good decisions depending on your own needs and budget.

Let's consider some of the elements important to doing your own contracting. This information can be modified to fit the needs of those hiring a contractor or doing all the work themselves.

First, you'll need plans and specifications for the job. Without these, subcontractors could not submit realistic bids. Written specifications will also help circumvent disagreements about how the job was to be done. A few sketches and a page or two of specifications may be adequate for a small job (Fig. 1-32); highly detailed blueprints are recommended for a big one. That's where the services of an architect come in handy.

Many experts suggest that you look for subcontractors who have at least five to ten years, experience in the business. Young subcontractors having somewhat less experience than that may be just as competent (and may be so eager to get your business that they'll reduce their fee).

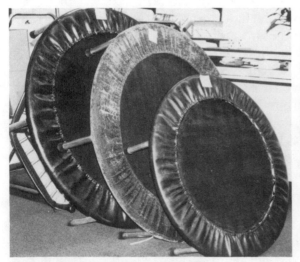

Fig. 1-26. Small trampolines or rebounders.

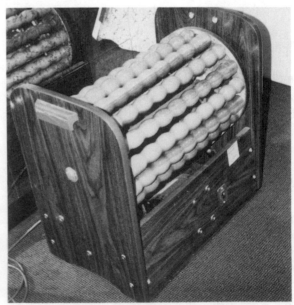

Fig. 1-27. Muscle tone machine.

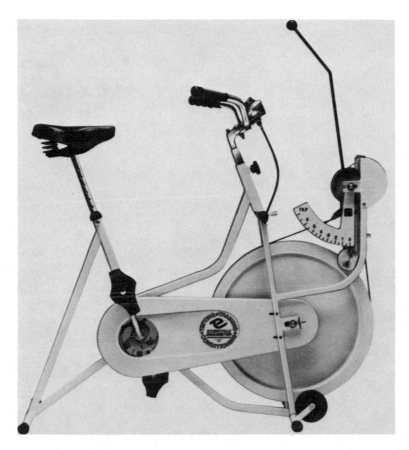

Fig. 1-28. Exercise
bicycle. (Courtesy Exercycle)

Ask friends, relatives, neighbors, your architect, home center personnel, and others in the home remodeling trades for the names of reputable subcontractors. Then ask those recommended subcontractors to give you names of homeowners for whom they have worked. If the subcontractors are proud of their work—and they should be—they'll be happy to provide such references.

When you check these references, ask each person the following questions:

☐ Were the subcontractors prompt?
☐ Did they do the work properly?
☐ Did they finish on time?
☐ Did they work within the agreed upon budget or did they bill you extra at the last minute?

☐ Did they return promptly when asked to correct mistakes?

Before hiring plumbers, electricians, and carpenters for your job, try to inspect a couple of projects each has done to see for yourself the kind of workmanship you can expect. You may not have the expertise to spot an extraordinarily good job, but you'll surely recognize a botched one when you see it.

You'll probably learn a great deal about the planned project and the skills it will require by discussing it with more than one subcontractor. Also, you might find a wide range between the highest and the lowest bids, and this could save you money. Don't pay more than you have to, but don't impulsively accept the lowest bid. Paying close to top dollar for a

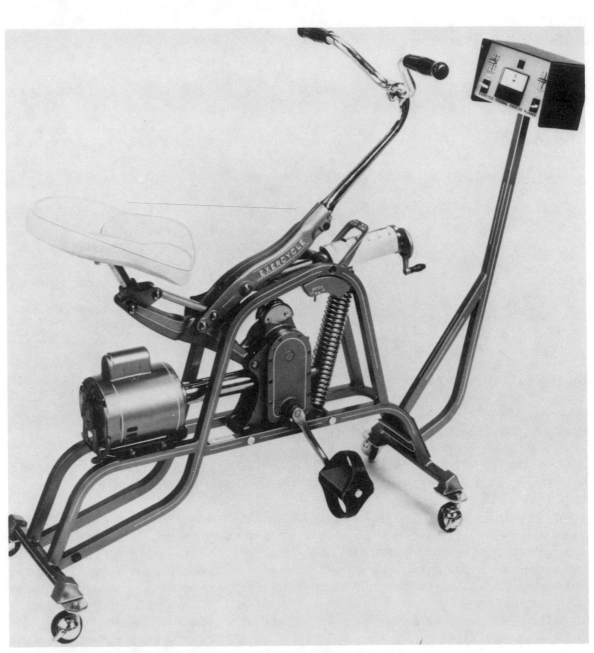

Fig. 1-29. Exercise bikes can be as fancy as you wish. (Courtesy Exercycle)

first-rate subcontractor may save you money in the long run.

FINANCING AND PAPERWORK

Contact several lenders and compare their interest rates, loan origination fees, and other financing costs. Also check on the pros and cons of refinancing your home mortgage. If you have an older mortgage, you may be able to refinance so that you pay a higher interest rate

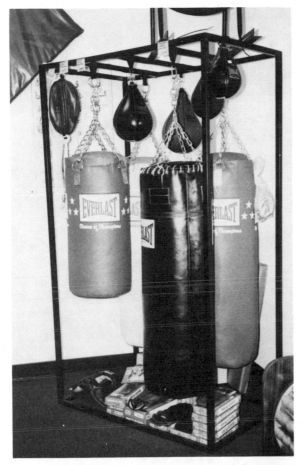

Fig. 1-30. Punching bags and body bags can also be installed in your fitness center.

cite the basic specifications, including such considerations as the sizes, types, models, brands, and prices of important products and materials (or the equivalent).

Include the following:

☐ Dates when the work will be started and completed (be firm here, but don't ask for the impossible).
☐ Warranties on workmanship (usually a year).
☐ Product warranties—as much as 10 to 15 years—provided by the manufacturer, with copies submitted by the subcontractor.
☐ Cleanup and debris removal provided by the subcontractor.

Also be sure to state that the costs and

on only the additional money you borrow. You may have to pay a fee to cover the cost of processing the new arrangement, however. Even if you can't refinance your mortgage this way, you may be able to bargain with the lender for a new rate that is lower than prevailing rates.

No matter how trustworthy a subcontractor may appear, accepting a verbal agreement is not wise. Such agreements are easily forgotten, leaving you open to potentially catastrophic misunderstandings.

The written agreement with each contractor, subcontractor, or craftsman should

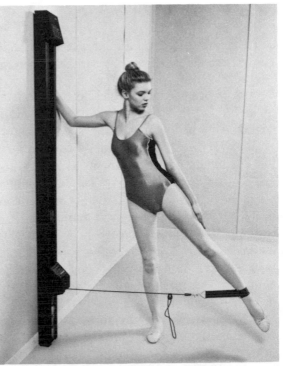

Fig. 1-31. A stress exerciser can be installed in a small amount of space. (Courtesy AMF)

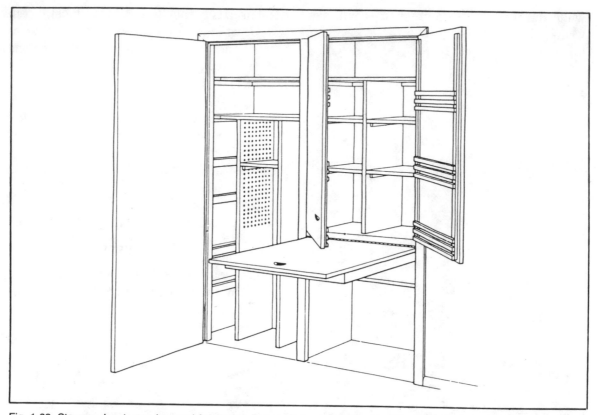

Fig. 1-32. Storage closets can be used for storing fitness equipment not in use. (Courtesy Georgia-Pacific)

details of any changes or additions made later must be put in writing. Spell out a specific schedule of payments. If the subcontractors request cash down payments, try to keep them low. Schedule partial payments to be made as the work progresses. A typical arrangement would have you pay 50 percent when the work is half done and the balance on completion. You may want to withhold 10 percent or so for up to 30 days after completion of the project, giving yourself time to look for mistakes. The unpaid amount will prompt the subcontractor to return promptly and correct them.

Resist the temptation to leave anything to chance. Only 16 states have laws that might protect you in case of problems, and according to the National Consumer Law Center, most of these laws are inadequate.

A building permit is usually required for making structural changes in a house, such as adding a room, carport, garage, or below-ground swimming pool or for installing new wiring or plumbing. The electrician or plumber ordinarily obtains these. Other types of remodeling may not require a permit. To find out whether one is required, call your community's building inspector.

INSURANCE

Each subcontractor hired should give you a certificate showing that he carries both *worker's compensation insurance* and *liability insurance*. The first type covers you if a worker is accidentally injured on your premises. The second covers you if any other person is injured or if your property is damaged while the work is in progress. You will also want to check with your own insurance agent to find out what liability and coverage you have toward subcontractors and workers.

A *mechanic's lien*, also called a materialman's lien, protects the supplier of building materials. In many states, an unpaid supplier can put a lien on your house to obtain payment from you, even though you paid the subcontractor who ordered the materials. Without insurance specifically covering mechanic's liens you can be forced to pay twice.

Laws regarding mechanic's liens differ from state to state. In New York State, for example, homeowners are protected if they have proof that they paid their subcontractor in full for the work ordered. In Louisiana and Hawaii, the law requires the subcontractor to provide homeowners with a bond, *if requested*, to protect them against such a lien.

Check with your state consumer protection bureau or your lawyer. If you're still confused, request that each subcontractor give you a "waiver of lien" and receipts showing that all suppliers have been paid before you make the final payment. Some subcontractors won't be able or willing to provide such legal papers. In that case, call the principal suppliers to make certain that each has been paid. As an alternative, arrange beforehand to pay the suppliers yourself and have the subcontractors deduct those payments from their bills. Doing your own contracting may not be easy, but it can be immensely satisfying.

DOING IT YOURSELF

You may decide to do the whole job yourself—large or small. In this case, you'll learn how to select and use common tools and see how easy it is to build fitness equipment and remodel or install fitness rooms. In the next chapter we will look at the tools and techniques for building your own fitness center.

2

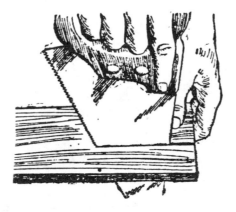

Tools and Techniques

BUILDING YOUR OWN FITNESS CENTER CAN BE easy—and even fun—if you know how to select and use common woodworking tools, materials, and fasteners. Whether you're a first-time or long-time do-it-yourselfer, you'll find both the tools and techniques in this chapter to make your fitness center more enjoyable to build and use.

Let's first take a look at the tools you'll need. You may have some of them on hand right now. Others may be rented or purchased as needed. It all depends upon your budget and how much you hope to use them in the future. A 10-inch radial arm saw may not be a good investment for cutting a few pieces of wood, but it can probably pay for itself if you're adding a fitness room in your home.

Tools can be broken down into two broad categories depending on what makes them operate: hand tools and power tools. We'll cover hand tools first, including hammers, hand-saws, screwdrivers, chisels, brace and bit, planes, files, measuring tools, miscellaneous tools, and sharpeners.

HAMMERS

The *claw hammer* (Fig. 2-1) is the backbone of any tool kit. Select one on the basis of its weight and balance. For small work, such as driving in tacks and brads, use an upholsterer's or tack hammer. The striking face of the hammer should be kept free of dirt and rust. This will prevent the face from slipping off the head of the nail and damaging the wood surface. A loose hammer head can be tightened by driving small metal wedges into the top of the handle. Soaking the hammer head in water to tighten it is only a temporary cure and not satisfactory. Do not use a claw hammer for prying up heavy planks or for pulling out heavy spikes as the claws will break.

To drive a nail straight, keep the face of

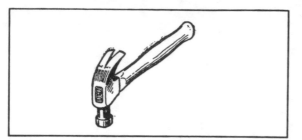

Fig. 2-1. Typical claw hammer.

the hammer head at the same angle as the head of the nail. By doing this you will avoid the natural tendency to strike the nailhead unevenly. Use sharp taps rather than heavy blows. This will give you more control over the hammer and you will hit the nailhead squarely.

HANDSAWS

There are two kinds of handsaws (Fig. 2-2): the *crosscut,* used for cutting across the grain of the wood, and the *ripsaw* for cutting with the grain. The teeth of a crosscut saw are triangular, the front of each tooth being filed to a 15-degree angle and the back to a 45-degree angle. The teeth are "set" or bent alternately

to one side or to the other. The teeth of a ripsaw are chisel shaped, the front of each tooth filed to an 8-degree angle and the rear to a 52-degree angle. The teeth of a ripsaw are "set" in the same fashion as those of the crosscut saw.

The size of a saw is measured by the number of points to the inch. The number of teeth to an inch is always one less than the number of points to the inch. A crosscut saw of average size is 8 points, while a ripsaw should be about 7 points.

Saws should be kept free of rust by wiping them with light oil after they have been used. Be very careful when sawing used lumber not to strike a nail or some metal object in the wood. This will dull the teeth to such a degree that the saw will be of little use until it has been sharpened. Do not try to work with a dull saw. This is too much of a handicap for even a skilled workman. Sharpening a saw properly requires skill and experience, and unless you are willing to devote considerable time to this job, it's best to have it sharpened by a professional.

Figure 2-3 illustrates a safe way to place a saw when not in use. Figure 2-4 offers the

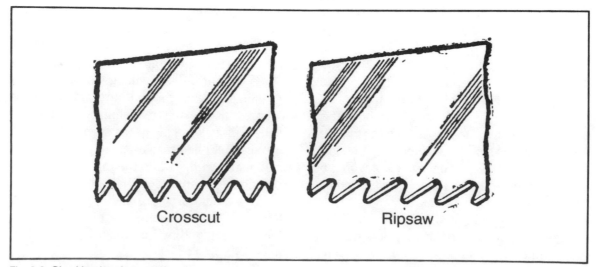

Fig. 2-2. Checking handsaw teeth.

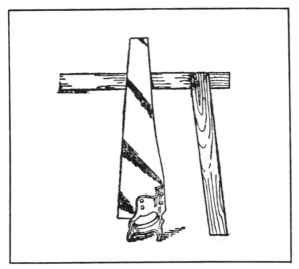

Fig. 2-3. Safe handsaw storage.

method of tightening the handle of a handsaw with screws.

To saw a straight line—not as easy as it might sound—just follow a few simple rules. First, the line to be cut should be marked using a square or rule so that the line will be straight. Don't trust your eye alone as a guide when sawing. By marking two or more sides of the wood before starting you provide additional assurance that the cut will be right.

Hold the saw at a 45-degree angle to the wood for crosscutting and at a 60-degree angle when ripping (Fig. 2-5). Use the knuckle of the thumb as a guide. A piece of wood can be used instead of the thumb and this will prevent injury in case the saw jumps. The first few strokes of the saw will indicate whether you are going to get a square cut or not. Saw with slow, deliberate strokes and don't hurry.

Figure 2-6 illustrates how to saw with the grain. Allow the saw to cut without applying any downward pressure on the blade. A small nail driven in the opening of the cut will prevent the wood from closing in on the saw and causing it to bind.

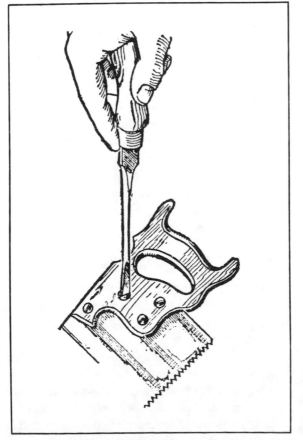

Fig. 2-4. Tightening handsaw blade and handle.

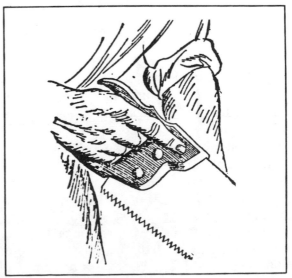

Fig. 2-5. Holding a handsaw.

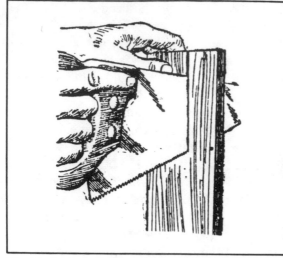
Fig. 2-6. Sawing with the grain.

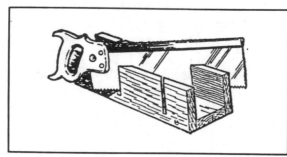
Fig. 2-7. Tenon saw with miter box.

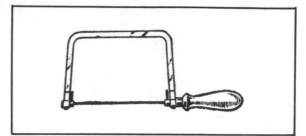
Fig. 2-8. Coping saw.

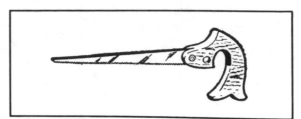
Fig. 2-9. Keyhole saw.

Figure 2-7 illustrates a *tenon saw,* also called a backsaw or miter saw. It is a crosscut saw with 12 to 16 points to the inch, a thin blade, and a reinforced back. This saw is used to make the very fine cuts required in cabinetwork and other fine woodwork. To make the cuts accurate, the tenon saw should be used in conjunction with a miter box.

The *coping saw* (Fig. 2-8) is used for fine work and for cutting curves in wood. The blade is held in the frame under tension and can be turned in the frame so that cuts may be made at different angles. The blades can be removed when they become dull or broken. Keep a sup-

ply of extra blades in the tool kit because thin blades are easily broken.

The blade of the *compass saw* or *keyhole saw* (Fig. 2-9) is pointed and is used primarily for cutting curves where it would be impossible to use a coping saw because of the frame. The general practice in working with the compass saw is to drill a hole with a brace and bit large enough for the blade of the saw. Once this is done, the saw is inserted in the hole and the remainder of the wood is cut out with the saw.

SCREWDRIVERS

A good tool kit should contain screwdrivers of various sizes. The most common types are the *flathead screwdriver* (Fig. 2-10 and the crosshead or *Phillips.*

Don't try to remove heavy screws with a screwdriver that is obviously too small. The screwdriver will slip out of the notch in the screw and damage the screwhead. There is also a considerable chance of twisting the handle loose from the blade.

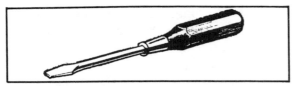

Fig. 2-10. Typical screwdriver.

A screwdriver eight inches long is about right for most heavy work found in the home. A three-inch screwdriver will be needed for small work and a long, thin one for electrical and other work in which the screws are relatively small and inaccessible.

Here's a common problem: don't use a screwdriver for any purpose other than turning screws. Screwdrivers used as cold chisels, pry bars, and the like cannot be expected to last long. Keep the blade of a screwdriver sharp. Use a file for this purpose rather than a grindstone. Grinding the blade of a screwdriver may overheat the metal and cause it to lose temper.

A *ratchet screwdriver* with interchangeable blades is an excellent time-saver on jobs that require a great many screws. This screwdriver does away with lifting the blade from the screw after every half-turn. Change the blades according to the size of the screws to be turned. A ratchet screwdriver requires a little light oiling now and then on all moving parts.

Occasionally you will run up against a screw which calls for a special screwdriver. These screws are mostly automobile and machine screws. Don't attempt to use a common screwdriver on them. A special screwdriver, made to fit the heads of these screws, should be used.

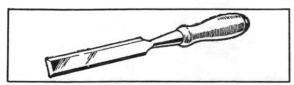

Fig. 2-11. Typical wood chisel.

CHISELS

There are many different kinds of wood chisels and gouges, but for general purposes the firmer chisel (Fig. 2-11) is the best suited for both light and heavy work. There are two classes of chisels: the *tang chisel* and the *socket chisel*. The names refer to the manner in which the blade is attached to the handle. The tang chisel has a sharply-pointed tang driven into the wood handle, while the handle of the socket chisel is driven into a socket at the end of the blade. Wood chisels are from ⅛ to 2 inches wide, but a ¼-inch, ½-inch, and a ¾-inch chisel will be sufficient for most jobs in this book.

Use a wood-head or rubber-head mallet for striking a chisel, never a hammer with a metal face. To preserve a good cutting edge on the chisels, the blades should not be allowed to come in contact with other tools or metal. Don't overstrain a chisel by trying to make too big a cut. Small cuts will give you more accuracy in your work, and the job will be done just as quickly in the long run.

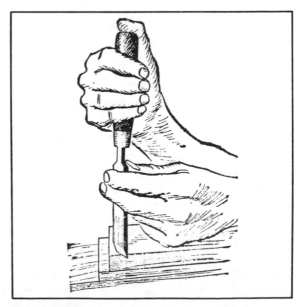

Fig. 2-12. Making a vertical cut with a wood chisel.

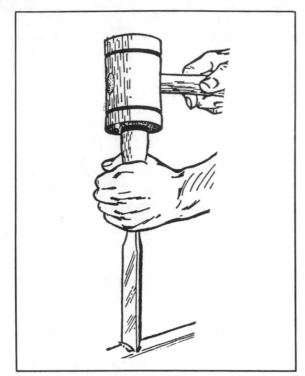

Fig. 2-13. Holding a wood chisel for a mallet.

Figure 2-12 illustrates how to hold a wood chisel when making a vertical cut. Figure 2-13 shows how to hold a chisel for striking with a mallet.

BRACE AND BIT

With the invention of the power drill, many shops have discarded the old brace and bit. Get one if you can as they offer precise drilling at a low cost. A *ratchet brace* (Fig. 2-14) is a device to hold wood-boring tools. The ratchet assembly allows this tool to be operated in a limited space where it would be impossible for the handle of the brace to make a complete revolution.

Auger bits come in many sizes and are measured by sixteenths of an inch, beginning with 3/16 inch. The number stamped on the tang of the bit indicates the size of the hole the

bit will make, measured in sixteenths of an inch. A bit stamped 8/16 would be a ½-inch bit.

The two main parts of a bit are the twist and the shank. The twist can be either single or double and terminates in two points. The points score the circle to be cut, while the two sharp edges do the actual cutting. The screw at the center pulls the bit into the wood as it turns.

When boring a vertical hole into a piece of wood, use a square to align the brace and bit with the wood. Once the bit is in the wood, it can be bent or broken if the position of the brace is suddenly changed. When boring deep holes it is a good idea to remove the bit from time to time to prevent any possibility of choking the hole with waste wood. Bits are self-cleaning and waste wood will move up along the twist of the bit and come out the top. But very often there is enough waste wood left in the hole to cause difficulty.

Don't try to make a hole right through a piece of wood. Bore through one side until the screw of the bit appears on the bottom side. Remove the bit, turn the wood over and place the screw of the bit in the opening made from the opposite side. By doing this you will avoid splintering the wood surface, which often occurs when the bit breaks through.

A device known as a *bit gauge* (Fig. 2-15) is used to prevent making a hole too deep. This tool is very handy to remove excess wood and is often necessary when making certain kinds

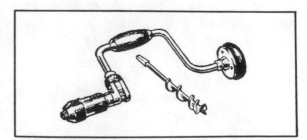

Fig. 2-14. Ratchet brace.

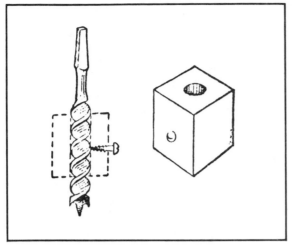

Fig. 2-15. Bit gauge.

of wood joints. The bit gauge fits over the bit and is then screwed on tightly at the proper depth for the hole. The same results can be obtained by drilling a hole in a block of wood and leaving the block on the bit. The width of the block will depend on the depth of the hole. The thicker the block, the shorter will be the portion of bit exposed for drilling.

An *expansion bit* (Fig. 2-16) is used for drilling holes larger than can be made with ordinary size bits. A *rose countersink* (Fig. 2-17) that can be fitted into the brace is used for boring conical holes to receive the heads of screws so that the head will be flush with the surface of the wood. *Forstner bits* (Fig. 2-18) are used in boring holes in thin wood or in end-grain wood. They have no twist and make a very accurate cut. To avoid any possibility of the wood's splitting, it's a good idea to start the hole with an auger bit and finish with a forstner bit.

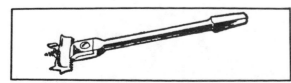

Fig. 2-16. Expansion bit.

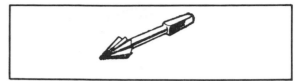

Fig. 2-17. Rose countersink.

Twist drills of the type used for drilling metal are made with a square shank to fit a wood brace. They are very useful for making small holes in wood, such as those needed for wood screws.

Screwdriver bits are also made to fit the brace. When used in a ratchet brace the same advantages are gained as with a ratchet screwdriver. However, driving down a screw so that it is straight is somewhat more difficult with a brace than with a ratchet screwdriver.

Keep all bits that have cutting edges free of contact with other tools. The moving parts of the brace should be oiled from time to time to keep them operating properly.

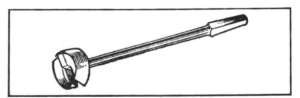

Fig. 2-18. Forstner bit.

The *hand drill* (Fig. 2-19) is an older style tool that can be used for making holes in either wood or metal, depending upon the kind of drill used. The tool made to fit a hand drill has a round shank instead of the square one used with a brace. The hand drill is excellent for making small and numerous holes in wood as it can be operated a great deal faster than a wood brace. Of course, it is not as fast as the more expensive electric drill. Both the wood and metal drills are relatively small in diameter. They can be bent or broken easily by running the drill too fast or moving the drill once it has penetrated the wood or metal.

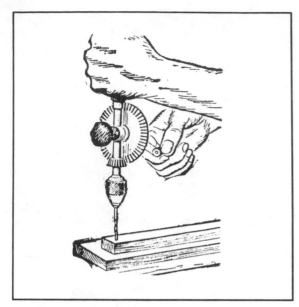

Fig. 2-19. Typical hand drill.

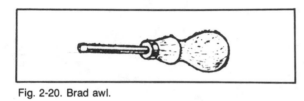

Fig. 2-20. Brad awl.

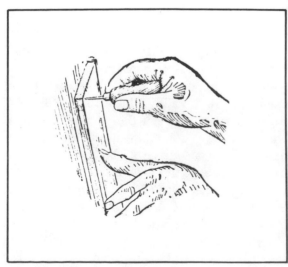

Fig. 2-21. Making a hole with a brad awl.

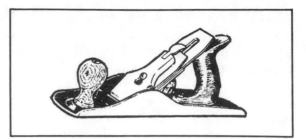

Fig. 2-22. Jack plane.

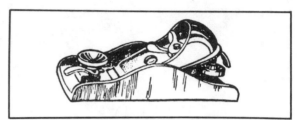

Fig. 2-23. Block plane.

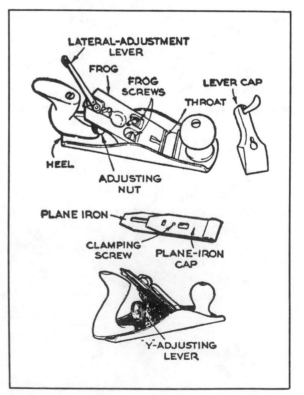

Fig. 2-24. Plane parts.

34

Figure 2-20 illustrates a related tool often used in woodworking, the *brad awl*. This small, wood-boring tool can be found in several sizes. It's used for drilling holes for screws and nails. In making a hole, the edge of the blade should be placed across the grain and then pressed into the wood and rotated slightly (Fig. 2-21). As the efficiency of this tool depends on a good cutting edge, it should receive the same care as the chisels and the wood bits.

PLANES

Planes can be found in many sizes and shapes, depending on the type of work to be done. For general purposes the *jack plane* (Fig. 2-22) is adequate. This plane is about 14 inches long and 2 inches wide. It is suitable for rough work but cannot produce a very smooth surface because its length will cause the blade to slip over the low spots.

When a greater degree of smoothness is required, a *smoothing plane,* somewhat shorter than the jack, is used. For small work and for end-grain planing, the block plane (Fig. 2-23) is used.

The *blade* or *plane iron* (Fig. 2-24) can be adjusted for depth by moving the knurled knob located at the back of the blade. The lateral adjustment of the blade is made with a lever that fits into a slot on the upper portion of the blade. The blade has a cap which fits over it to provide additional strength. On hard-grain wood, or for crossplaning, this cap should be set as close to the edge as possible. This will prevent the wood from splintering. A block plane doesn't have this cap as it is designed for end-grain planing.

The first rule in planing is to work in the direction of the grain (Fig. 2-25). This direction can be determined with the first stroke. If the blade tears the wood and makes a rough surface, reverse the direction and work from the other end. Don't try to take off too much wood at one time. Set the blade so that a thin shaving will be taken off rather than large chunks of wood. If you do this you will get greater accuracy and a smooth surface. Figure 2-26 illustrates how to guide the plane with your left hand.

FILES

A *wood file* is used in smoothing wood that is difficult or impossible to work with other tools. Files are classified according to their length, shape, and the spacing of the teeth. A file used for rough work is called a rasp. A metal file is very useful for sharpening screwdrivers and other tools. Both wood and metal files should be fitted with handles to avoid injury to the hands. Figure 2-27 depicts a typical file, the half-round.

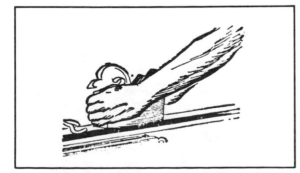

Fig. 2-25. Planing in the direction of the grain.

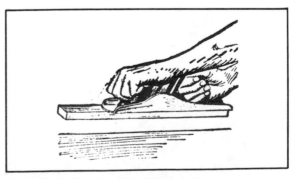

Fig. 2-26. Guiding the plane with the left hand.

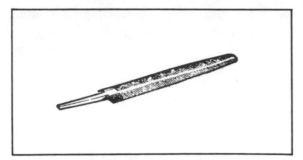

Fig. 2-27. Half-round file.

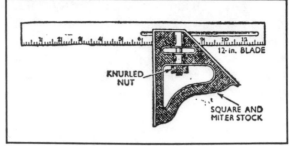

Fig. 2-29. Combination or try square.

MEASURING TOOLS

You cannot build your fitness center without the aid of at least one type of measuring tool. Let's take a quick look at the more common ones.

The retractable *tape measure* is extremely handy while being highly accurate for measuring everything from fitness equipment parts to wall stud placement. Common lengths include 6 feet, 12 feet, and 20 feet, with longer and shorter units available. Invest in the longest and best quality tape measure you can afford.

A large 24-by-16-inch *steel framing square* (Fig. 2-28) can be used on numerous jobs. Besides the scale of inches and a right angle, it can be used for laying out many other angles. Don't allow the steel square to become rusty as it will make accurate readings difficult.

A *try square* (Fig. 2-29) is somewhat smaller with a wood or metal handle. It has many uses in the home workshop, such as

making angles and squaring off small pieces of wood. The *combination square* can be used to lay out 90-degree and 45-degree angles. Many of these squares have a level built into the handle.

To check any piece of work to be sure that it is either horizontal or vertical, a *level* is needed. A level has a small tube filled with water in which a small bubble of air floats. The tube is marked off so that the level is either vertical or horizontal when the bubble of air is centered between the lines on the tube. Figure 2-30 shows a typical level.

OTHER HAND TOOLS

There are numerous other hand tools that can help you build and install your fitness center. A *nail set* (Fig. 2-31) is a small tool used to drive the heads of nails below the surface of the wood. A tool kit should contain at least two nail sets, one for large nails and the other for small.

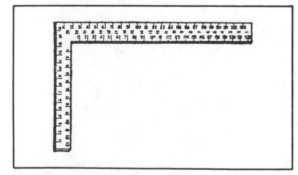

Fig. 2-28. Steel framing square.

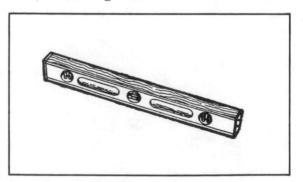

Fig. 2-30. Typical carpenter's level.

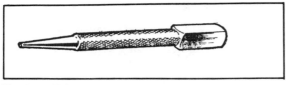
Fig. 2-31. Nail set.

The wide, thin blade of the *putty knife* (Fig. 2-32) is necessary for glazing and such work as installing drywall. Keep the blade clean and free of rust.

A pair of *adjustable pliers* (Fig. 2-33) is one of the most useful tools in your kit. It can be used for tightening small machine nuts, bending wire, and many other odd jobs. A set of *wrenches* or *sockets* will also be useful in assembling equipment for your fitness center.

POWER TOOLS

The variety of power tools for the builder and woodworker seems to grow each year. Most are based on the hand tools covered in the first segment of this chapter, however. They include power saws, shaving tools, lathes, drill presses, and related tools. Since there are so many variations and combinations to these power tools, we'll take a broad look at the types and uses.

SAWS

Mechanical woodworking saws range in size and power from small shop jigsaws to huge bandsaws. Most fit into the circular saw family.

The *circular saw* has a blade which is mounted on, and spun by, a shaft called an arbor. Like a handsaw, a circular saw blade may be a crosscut saw or a ripsaw. The teeth of these saw blades are similar to those on the corresponding handsaws, and they cut on the same principle. A third type of circular saw blade, called a combination or miter saw blade, may be used for either crosscutting or ripping.

A *tilt-arbor bench*—commonly called a *table saw*—includes the blade and arbor/motor within the table. Its saw blade can be tilted for cutting bevels and the like by tilting the arbor. For ripping stock, the cutoff gauges are removed, and the ripping fence is set a distance away from the saw which is equal to the desired width of the piece to be ripped off. The piece is placed with one edge against the fence and fed through with the fence as a guide.

For cutting stock off square, the cutoff gauge is set at 90 degrees to the line of the saw, and the ripping fence is set to the outside edge of the table away from the stock to be cut. The piece is then placed with one edge against the cutoff gauge, held firmly, and fed through by pushing the gauge along its slot.

For safety, don't use a ripsaw for crosscutting or a crosscut saw for ripping. Also, check your saw over before turning it on. Make sure the blade is sharp, unbroken, and

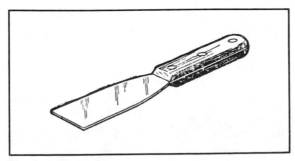
Fig. 2-32. Putty knife.

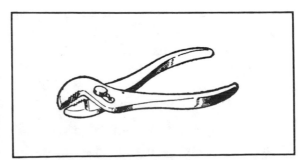
Fig. 2-33. Adjustable pliers.

free from cracks. Stand to one side of the saw rather than in front of it as you work so that a "kickback" will not throw stock into you.

A *radial arm saw* includes a motor and arbor pivoted on a yoke which can be swung in any direction. The yoke slides back and forth on an arm or overarm. The radial arm saw is adaptable to almost any conceivable type of saw cutting and is one of the most versatile power tools you can buy.

The portable electric *circular saw* is a great labor-saving device in sawing wood framing members on the job. By adding a ripping guide to your portable saw you can improve its accuracy and usefulness.

While the *bandsaw* is designed primarily for making curved cuts, it can also be used for straight cutting. Unlike the circular saws, the bandsaw is frequently used for freehand cutting. The bandsaw has two large wheels on which a continuous narrow saw blade or band turns, just as a belt is turned on pulleys. The saw blade is guided and kept in line by two sets of blade guides. Tensioning of the blade— tightening and loosening—is provided by another adjustment located just back of the upper wheel.

The size of a bandsaw is designed by the diameter of the wheels. Common sizes are 14, 16, 18, 20, 30, 36, 42, and 48 inches. Blades or bands for bandsaws are designated by points (tooth points per inch), thickness (gauge), and width.

A *jigsaw* performs about the same function as a bandsaw but is usually capable of cutting more intricate curves. Instead of a flexible band-type blade, the jigsaw has a short, straight rigid blade which is rapidly oscillated vertically by the power mechanism.

SHAVING TOOLS

To get the smooth surface or edge desired on certain materials, various operations must be

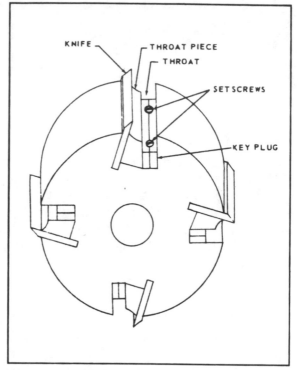

Fig. 2-34. Jointer cutterhead.

performed with shaving tools such as jointers, surfacers, and shapers. The *jointer* is a machine for power-planing stock on faces, edges, and ends. The planing is done by a revolving cutterhead equipped with two or more knives as shown in Fig. 2-34. The size of a jointer is designated by the width in inches of the cutterhead. Sizes range from 4 inches to 36 inches.

The principle on which the jointer functions is illustrated in Fig. 2-35. The table consists of two parts on either side of the cutterhead. The stock is started on the infeed table and fed past the cutterhead onto the outfeed table. The surface of the outfeed table must be exactly level with the highest point reached by the knife edges. The surface of the infeed table is lower by an amount equal to the desired depth of the cut.

A *single surfacer* or planer surfaces stock

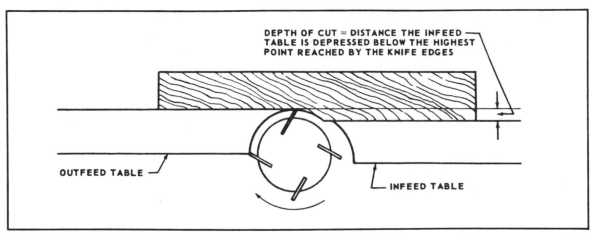

DEPTH OF CUT = DISTANCE THE INFEED
TABLE IS DEPRESSED BELOW THE HIGHEST
POINT REACHED BY THE KNIFE EDGES

OUTFEED TABLE

INFEED TABLE

Fig. 2-35. Operation of jointer.

on one face only, while a double surfacer surfaces both top and bottom surface. It operates
much like the jointer and is usually not found in
home workshops.

The *shaper* is designed primarily for edging curved stock and for cutting ornamental
edges such as on moldings. The flat cutter or
knives on a shaper are mounted on a vertical
spindle and held in place by a spindle nut. Refer
to Fig. 2-36 for a closer look at how the shaper
works. Figure 2-37 shows some common
shaper knives. Portable routers common to
many home workshops are actually shapers
and can be used to add beauty to the function of
your fitness center.

LATHES

The *lathe* is one of the oldest of all woodworking tools. The lathe is used in turning or shap-
ing round billets, drums, disks, and any object
that requires a true diameter. The size of a
lathe is determined by the maximum diameter
of the work it can swing over its bed. In lathe
work, wood is rotated against special cutting
tools which include turning gouges; skew
chisels; parting tools; round-nose, square-
nose and spear-point chisels; toothing irons;

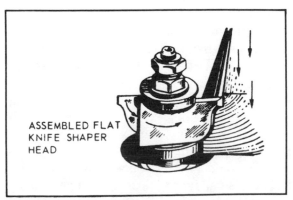

ASSEMBLED FLAT
KNIFE SHAPER
HEAD

Fig. 2-36. Operation of shaper.

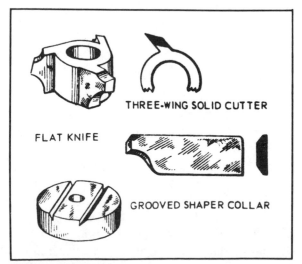

THREE-WING SOLID CUTTER

FLAT KNIFE

GROOVED SHAPER COLLAR

Fig. 2-37. Shaper knives.

39

and aids such as calipers, dividers, and templates.

Lathe turning may be divided into two categories: center-to-center turning or spindle turning and faceplate turning. A lathe can make decorative legs and supports for fitness equipment or be used to turn special pieces for gym or exercise equipment.

DRILL PRESS

A *drill press* is a stationary drilling machine often used for woodworking requiring numerous and exact holes. It always uses a twist drill rather than an auger bit for boring.

PORTABLE DRILLS

Portable drills are very popular with woodworkers as the portable drill offers help with a number of jobs at a relatively low cost. Capacity of the drill is measured by chuck size. Also, since speed and power are directly related to capacity, the bigger the drill you buy, the more power it will have and the slower its speed. Slower speeds are required for heavier operations.

Check with your hardware store, describing the uses you will have for your portable drill. They can help you size and use your machine correctly.

SANDERS

Many do-it-yourselfers invest in sanders, though they are not necessary for most fitness center projects. Sanding requirements is minimal. If you do want a sander, you can choose between a stationary or portable model. The stationary sander, of course, costs more and needs greater use to pay for itself.

There are two types of sanders: belt and disc. A *belt sander* rotates a continuous belt of special sandpaper much as a bandsaw rotates a blade, except on a smaller scale. A *disc sander* uses a circular disc of sandpaper rotated by a drill. A disc sander can do finer sanding on smaller jobs. A belt sander is better for larger flat surfaces.

FASTENERS

Fasteners attach one element to another. Simple enough; however, there are all types and sizes of fasteners: nails, screws, bolts, glue, and others. In the coming pages, you'll learn about the more common fasteners you'll use to build your fitness center.

NAILS

The standard nail used in woodworking and home construction is the *wire nail,* so called because it is made from wire. There are many types of nails classified according to use and form. The wire nail is round-shafted, straight, pointed, and may vary in size, weight, size and shape of head, type of point, and finish.

Before covering the many types of nails further, consider some basic rules for selecting and using nails. First, whatever the type, a nail should be at least three times as long as the thickness of wood it is intended to hold. Two-thirds of the length of the nail is driven into the second piece for proper anchorage, while one-third provides the necessary anchorage of the piece being fastened. Nails should be driven at an angle slightly toward each other and should be carefully placed to provide the greatest holding power.

Common wire nails and box nails are the same except that the wire sizes are one or two numbers smaller for a given length of box nail than they are for the common nail. The common wire nail (Fig. 2-38) is used for housing construction framing. The common wire nail and the box nail are generally used for structural construction.

The *finishing nail* is made from finer wire and has a smaller head than the common nail. It may be set below the surface of the wood and

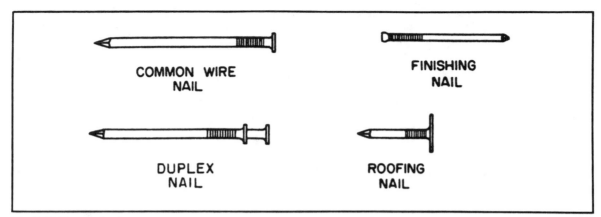

Fig. 2-38. Types of nails.

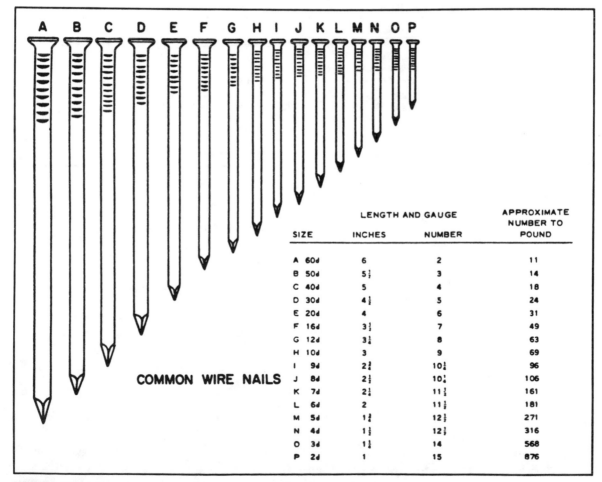

COMMON WIRE NAILS

SIZE	LENGTH AND GAUGE		APPROXIMATE NUMBER TO POUND
	INCHES	NUMBER	
A 60d	6	2	11
B 50d	$5\frac{1}{2}$	3	14
C 40d	5	4	18
D 30d	$4\frac{1}{2}$	5	24
E 20d	4	6	31
F 16d	$3\frac{1}{2}$	7	49
G 12d	$3\frac{1}{4}$	8	63
H 10d	3	9	69
I 9d	$2\frac{3}{4}$	$10\frac{1}{4}$	96
J 8d	$2\frac{1}{2}$	$10\frac{1}{4}$	106
K 7d	$2\frac{1}{4}$	$11\frac{1}{2}$	161
L 6d	2	$11\frac{1}{2}$	181
M 5d	$1\frac{3}{4}$	$12\frac{1}{2}$	271
N 4d	$1\frac{1}{2}$	$12\frac{1}{2}$	316
O 3d	$1\frac{1}{4}$	14	568
P 2d	1	15	876

Fig. 2-39. Nail sizes.

Table 2-1. Nail Size, Type, and Use.

Size	Lgth (in.)	Diam (in.)	Remarks	Where used
2d	1	.072	Small head	Finish work, shop work.
2d	1	.072	Large flathead	Small timber, wood shingles, lathes.
3d	1¼	.08	Small head	Finish work, shop work.
3d	1¼	.08	Large flathead	Small timber, wood shingles, lathes.
4d	1½	.098	Small head	Finish work, shop work.
4d	1½	.098	Large flathead	Small timber, lathes, shop work.
5d	1¾	.098	Small head	Finish work, shop work.
5d	1¾	.098	Large flathead	Small timber, lathes, shop work.
6d	2	.113	Small head	Finish work, casing, stops, etc., shop work.
6d	2	.113	Large flathead	Small timber, siding, sheathing, etc., shop work.
7d	2¼	.113	Small head	Casing, base, ceiling, stops, etc.
7d	2¼	.113	Large flathead	Sheathing, siding, subflooring, light framing.
8d	2½	.131	Small head	Casing, base, ceiling, wainscot, etc., shop work.
8d	2½	.131	Large flathead	Sheathing, siding, subflooring, light framing, shop work.
8d	1¼	.131	Extra-large flathead	Roll roofing, composition shingles.
9d	2¾	.131	Small head	Casing, base, ceiling, etc.
9d	2¾	.131	Large flathead	Sheathing, siding, subflooring, framing, shop work.
10d	3	.148	Small head	Casing, base, ceiling, etc., shop work.
10d	3	.148	Large flathead	Sheathing, siding, subflooring, framing, shop work.
12d	3¼	.148	Large flathead	Sheathing, subflooring, framing.
16d	3½	.162	Large flathead	Framing, bridges, etc.
20d	4	.192	Large flathead	Framing, bridges, etc.
30d	4½	.207	Large flathead	Heavy framing, bridges, etc.
40d	5	.225	Large flathead	Heavy framing, bridges, etc.
50d	5½	.244	Large flathead	Extra-heavy framing, bridges, etc.
60d	6	.262	Large flathead	Extra-heavy framing, bridges, etc.

¹ This chart applies to wire nails, although it may be used to determine the length of cut nails.

will leave only a small hole which can be easily puttied up. It is generally used for interior or exterior finishing work and is used for finished carpentry and cabinetmaking.

The *duplex nail* is made with what appears to be two heads. The reason for this design is that the duplex nail is not meant to be permanent. It is used in the construction of temporary structures such as scaffolding and forms for foundations.

Roofing nails are round-shaped, diamond-pointed, galvanized nails of relatively short length and comparatively large heads. They are designed for fastening flexible roofing materials and for resisting continuous exposure to weather.

Nail sizes are designated by the use of the term "penny," such as 16-penny or 16d nail.

The wire gauge number varies according to type. Figure 2-39 illustrates the sizing of nails and approximate number of nails to the pound. Table 2-1 gives the general size and type of nail preferred for most applications.

SCREWS

Selecting screws over nails as fasteners depends on the type of material being fastened, the strength required, the finished appearance needed, and other factors. Using screws is more expensive than using nails. Screw sizes and dimensions are shown in Table 2-2.

The common *wood screw* is usually made of unhardened steel, stainless steel, aluminum, or brass. The steel may be bright finished or blued, zinc, cadmium, or chrome plated. Wood screws are threaded from a gimlet point of about two-thirds of the length of the screw and have a slotted head designed to be driven by inserting a screwdriver.

Wood screws (Fig. 2-40) are designated according to head style. The most common are: flathead, ovalhead, and roundhead, both in slotted and Phillips heads. To prepare wood for receiving the screws, bore a pilot hole the diameter of the screw to be used in the piece of wood. Some screws are countersunk to permit a covering material to cover the head (Fig. 2-41).

Lag screws or lag bolts are longer and much heavier than the common wood screw. They have coarser threads which extend from a cone or gimlet point slightly more than half the length of the screw.

Sheet metal screws are used for assembling metal parts. These screws are made regularly in steel and brass with four types of heads: flat, round, oval, and fillister.

BOLTS

Bolts are used in construction when great strength is required or when the work must be frequently disassembled. They usually use nuts for fastening and sometimes require washers to protect the surface of the material they are used to fasten. Figure 2-42 illustrates the common types of bolts available for fastening: carriage, machine, stove, and expansion.

Carriage bolts fall into three categories: square neck, finned neck, and ribbed neck. These bolts have roundheads that are not designed to be driven. They are threaded only part of the way up the shaft. Carriage bolts are chiefly for wood-to-wood applications.

Machine bolts are made with cut National Fine or National Coarse threads extending in length from twice the diameter of the bolt plus ¼ inch to twice the diameter plus ½ inch. They

Table 2-2. Screw Size and Dimensions.

Length (in.)	Size numbers																					
	0	1	2	3	4	5	6	7	8	9	10	11	12	13	14	15	16	17	18	20	22	24
1/4	x	x	x	x																		
3/8	x	x	x	x	x	x	x	x	x	x												
1/2			x	x	x	x	x	x	x	x	x	x	x									
5/8		x	x	x	x	x	x	x	x	x	x	x	x		x							
3/4			x	x	x	x	x	x	x	x	x	x	x		x		x					
7/8			x	x	x	x	x	x	x	x	x	x	x		x		x					
1				x	x	x	x	x	x	x	x	x	x		x		x		x	x		
1 1/4						x	x	x	x	x	x	x	x		x		x		x	x		x
1 1/2						x	x	x	x	x	x	x	x		x		x		x	x		x
1 3/4							x	x	x	x	x	x	x		x		x		x	x		x
2							x	x	x	x	x	x	x		x		x		x	x		x
2 1/4							x	x	x	x	x	x	x		x		x		x	x		x
2 1/2							x	x	x	x	x	x	x		x		x		x	x		x
2 3/4								x	x	x	x	x	x		x		x		x	x		x
3								x	x	x	x	x	x		x		x		x	x		x
3 1/2									x	x	x	x	x		x		x		x	x		x
4									x	x	x	x	x		x		x		x	x		x
4 1/2													x		x		x		x	x		x
5													x		x		x		x	x		x
6															x		x		x	x		x
Threads per inch	32	28	26	24	22	20	18	16	15	14	13	12	11		10		9		8	8		7
Diameter of screw (in.)	.060	.073	.086	.099	.112	.125	.138	.151	.164	.177	.190	.203	.216		.242		.268		.294	.320		.372

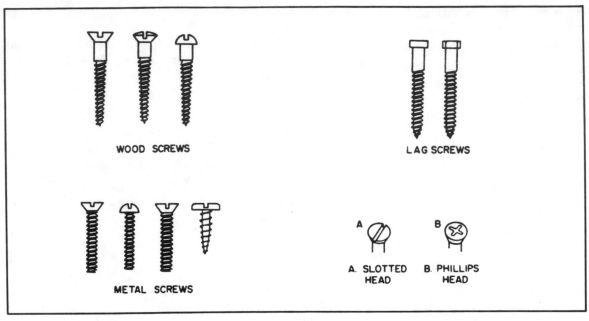

Fig. 2-40. Types of screws.

are precision made and generally applied metal-to-metal.

Stove bolts are less precisely made than machine bolts. They are made with either flat or round slotted heads and may have threads extending over the full length of the body, over part of the body, or over most of the body. They are generally used with square units and applied metal-to-metal, wood-to-wood, or wood-to-metal. If flatheaded, they are countersunk; if roundheaded, they are drawn flush to the surface.

An *expansion bolt* is used with an expansion shield to provide anchorage in substances in which a threaded fastener alone is useless, such as attaching a piece of equipment or frame to a drywall panel. *Corrugated fasteners* (Fig. 2-43) can be used to fasten joints and splices in small timber and boards.

GLUE

One of the oldest materials used for fastening is glue. There are several classes of glue including animal, fish, vegetable, casein, blood

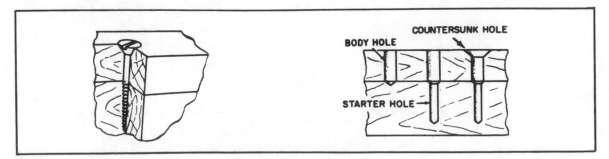

Fig. 2-41. Sinking screws properly.

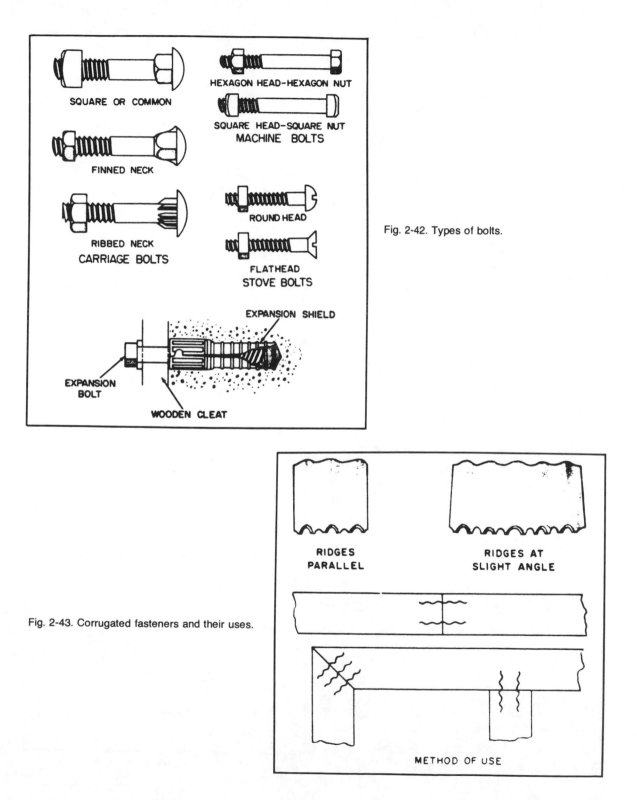

Fig. 2-42. Types of bolts.

Fig. 2-43. Corrugated fasteners and their uses.

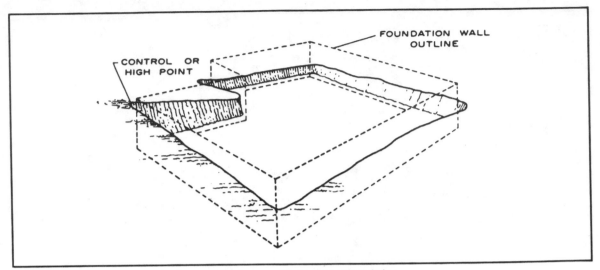

Fig. 2-44. Establishing the depth of excavation for your fitness center foundation.

albumin, and plastic resin. Each type of glue must be prepared and used in a special manner if you are to get the strongest possible joint. Instructions are found on the container label. Study these carefully before you attempt to use the glue.

There are also certain general principles which you should follow when you apply glue. A lot depends on the wood itself. Dry wood makes stronger joints than wood which is not well seasoned. This is easy to understand if you remember that water in the wood will decrease the amount of glue which can be absorbed.

UNDERSTANDING HOME CONSTRUCTION

To help you in planning and building your fitness center, let's discuss and illustrate the basic elements of home construction. Then you can better understand the more important components of the home that houses your fitness center and can more easily add to or remodel it.

The *footing* is located at the base of the foundation (Figs. 2-44 through 2-48). It is made of concrete and is considerably wider than the actual foundation. This is done so that the weight of the house will be distributed over a greater area. If the footing is not the right size for the weight of the house and the soil conditions, it will sink, and the house will tend to settle.

The *foundation* (Fig. 2-49) is the masonry on top of the footing and supports the weight of the house. It also provides the walls for the basement. The foundation can be made of stone, cement, cinder blocks, poured con-

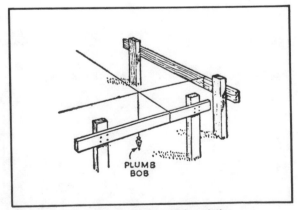

Fig. 2-45. Batter boards for a small foundation.

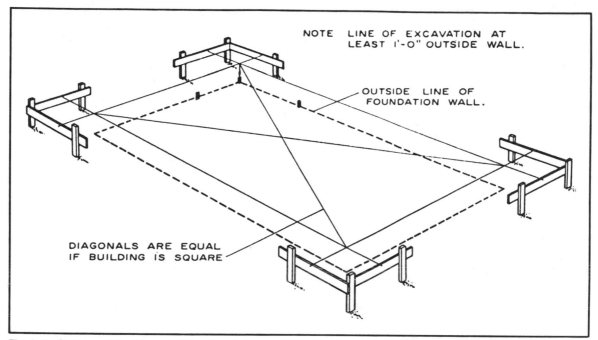

Fig. 2-46. Staking out the fitness building foundation.

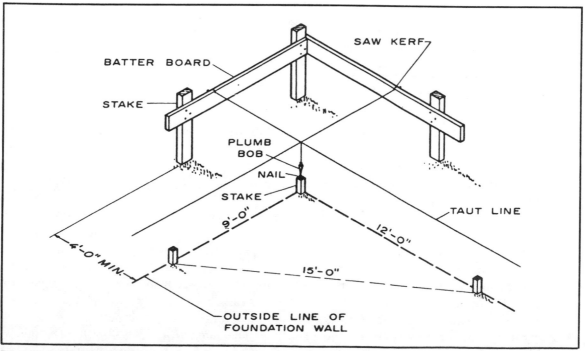

Fig. 2-47. Layout of excavation.

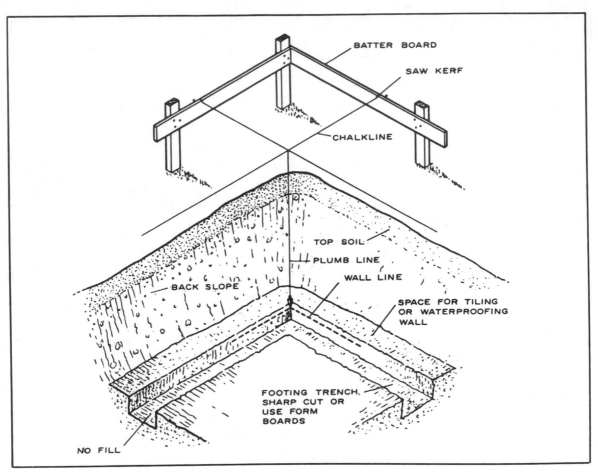

Fig. 2-48. Establishing corners and footings.

crete, or any other material that can sustain a considerable load.

Sills are the heavy wood or steel beams around the top of the foundation. These beams are attached and the house is built up from them. *Girders* are large beams running between opposite sills. They are used to provide additional support for the frame of the house as well as carry the flooring.

Floor joists are the beams that run across the sill and provide a base for the flooring. Floor joists are generally made of 2-×-10-inch or 2-×-8-inch lumber depending on the distance they must run. They are placed broad-

side upright for greater strength and, in well-constructed homes, are spaced sixteen inches from center to center.

Bridging consists of small strips of smaller lumber which are nailed diagonally between the floor joists along the center of the span. The purpose of the bridging is to keep the joists perpendicular so they will provide the maximum amount of support and to distribute the weight on the floor between several joists rather than one or two. Bridging can also be made out of strips of metal.

The *subflooring* (Fig. 2-50) is the under-flooring to which the finish floor is nailed or

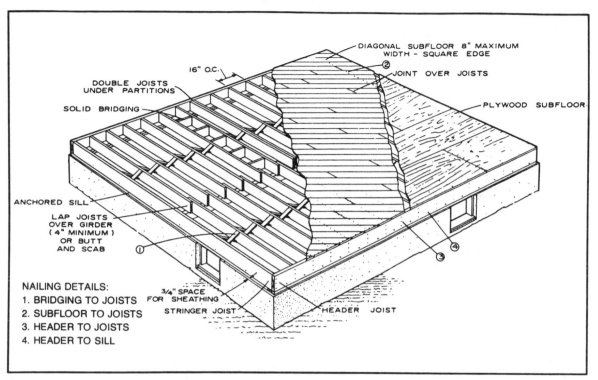

Fig. 2-49. Typical floor framing: (1) bridging, (2) subflooring, (3) header, (4) sill.

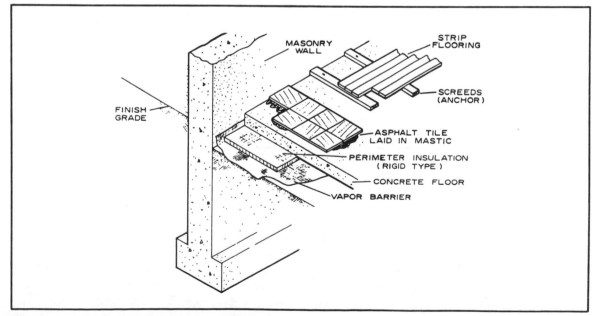

Fig. 2-50. Basement floor details for new construction.

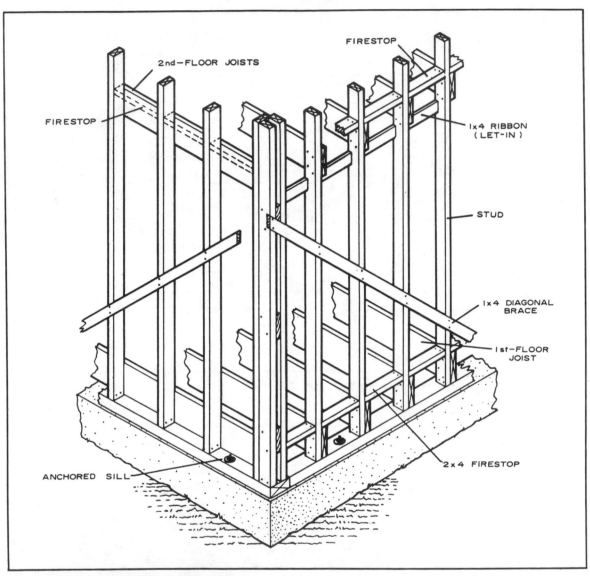

Fig. 2-51. Typical wall framing and components.

otherwise attached. The subfloor is nailed directly to the floor joists and runs either at a 45-degree or a 90-degree angle to them. The subfloor, or rough floor, not only furnishes a base for the finish floor but also adds a degree of strength to the frame of the house.

Studdings (Fig. 2-51) are the 2-×-4-inch upright timbers which act as supports for the walls. Studding is placed either 16 or 24 inches from center to center and is braced with diagonals, a protection against fire as the diagonals prevent the interior of the wall from becoming a flue. Horizontal pieces of studding are also nailed between the vertical studding at floor levels. These are called solid bridging. At each of the corners of a house is a 4-×-4-inch or

50

a double 2-×-4-inch timber used to provide additional support. Studding around window and door frames is also doubled. Interior wall surfaces are then attached to the studding.

Sheathing (Fig. 2-52) is generally made of tongue-and-grooved lumber nailed to the studding to form a portion of the exterior wall. Paneling is also used. After the sheathing has been put on, building paper is placed over it, and the outside wall of wood, brick, or stucco is raised. Sheathing provides additional strength for the frame of the house and is added protection against the wind and rain. Composition

board can also be used for sheathing.

Rafters (Fig. 2-53) for the roof are either 2 × 4s or 2 × 6s depending upon the size of the roof. If the roof has a composition shingle roofing, the entire roof is boarded over with sheathing (Fig. 2-54). If the roofing is made of wood shingles, shingle laths are nailed to the rafters to provide a base for the shingles. The *roof saddle* is made of two boards nailed together to form a V and placed over the top of the roof to cover the joint between the shingles. A *flashing* is a sheet of metal used for all joints on the exterior of the house formed by

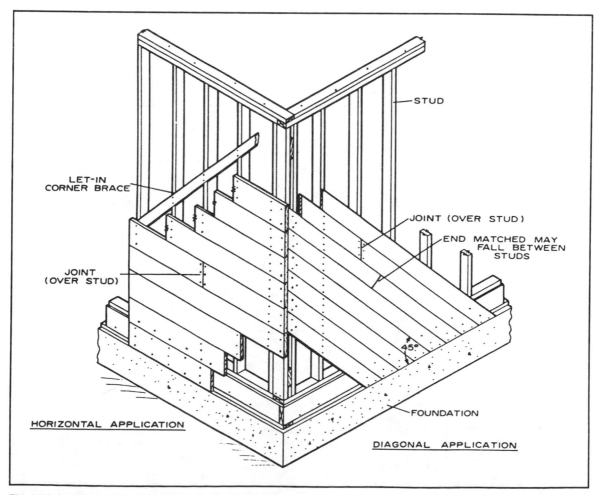

Fig. 2-52. Installing horizontal and diagonal wall sheathing.

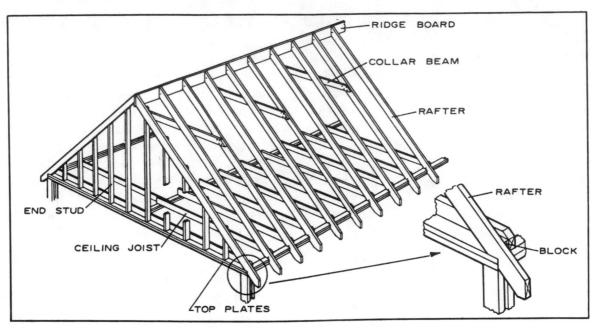

Fig. 2-53. Components of ceiling and roof framing.

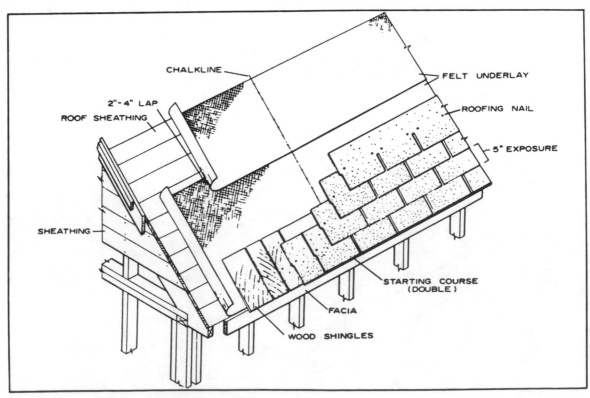

Fig. 2-54. Installing asphalt strip shingles or "tabs."

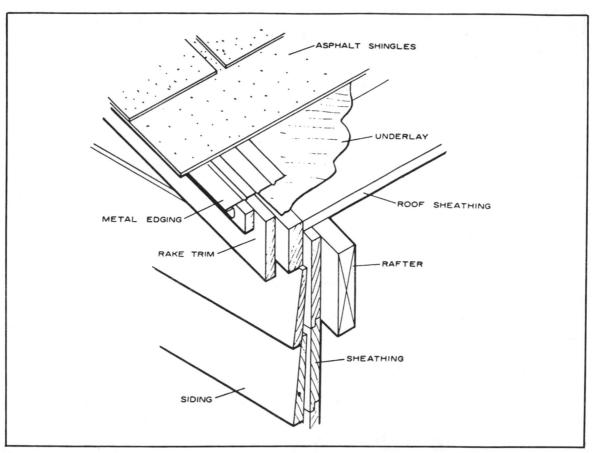

Fig. 2-55. Installing metal edging on a roof.

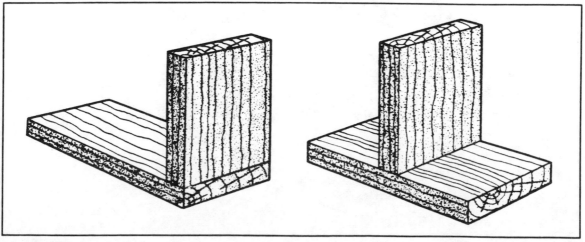

Fig. 2-56. Butt joints.

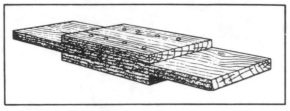

Fig. 2-57. End butt joints.

two different materials coming together or by angles in the roof (Fig. 2-55).

WOODWORKING

Constructing fitness equipment from wood requires an understanding of woodworking. There are many good books on this subject so we will cover only the basics you will need for the projects in this book.

The basic skill in woodworking is the art of joining pieces of wood to form tight, strong, well-made joints. Simple joints like the *butt* (Figs. 2-56 and 2-57), the *lap* joints (Fig. 2-58), and the *miter* joints (Fig. 2-59) are used mostly in rough or finish carpentry, though they may also be used occasionally in millwork and furniture making. More complex joints like the *rabbet* joints (Fig. 2-60), the *dado* and *gain* joints (Fig. 2-61), the *mortise-and-tenon* and *slip tenon* joints (Fig. 2-62), the *box corner* joints (Fig. 2-63), and the *dovetail* joints (Fig. 2-64) are used mostly in furniture, cabinet, and mill work.

To illustrate how joints play an important part in furniture construction, Fig. 2-65 illustrates the details of a typical cabinet. From this

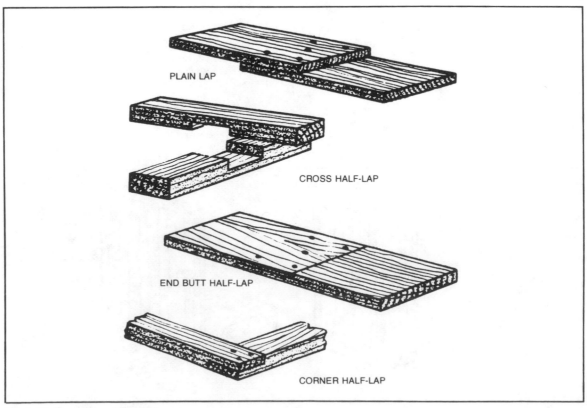

PLAIN LAP

CROSS HALF-LAP

END BUTT HALF-LAP

CORNER HALF-LAP

Fig. 2-58. Four types of lap joints.

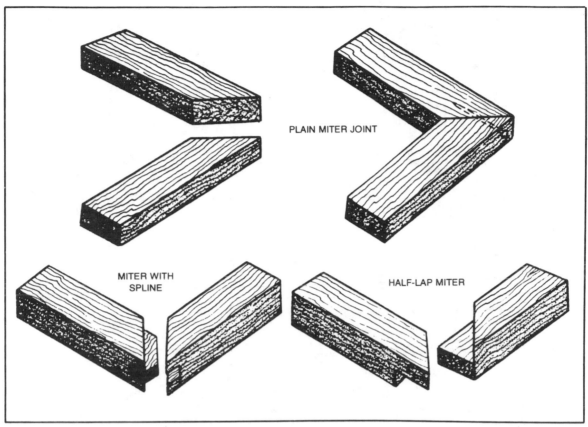

Fig. 2-59. Three types of miter joints.

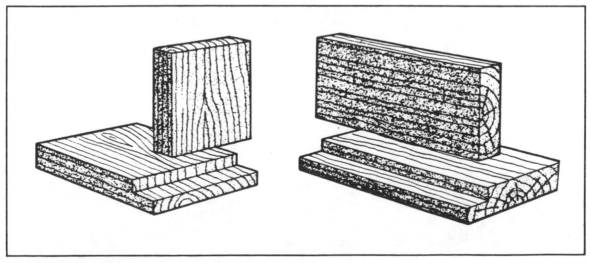

Fig. 2-60. Rabbet joints.

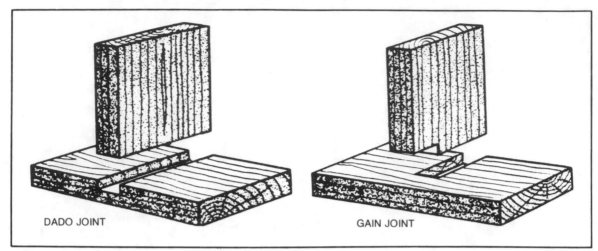

DADO JOINT   GAIN JOINT

Fig. 2-61. Dado and gain joints.

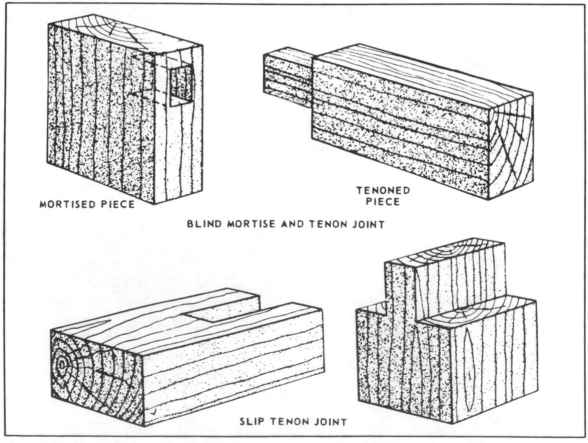

MORTISED PIECE   TENONED PIECE

BLIND MORTISE AND TENON JOINT

SLIP TENON JOINT

Fig. 2-62. Mortise-and-tenon and slip-tenon joints.

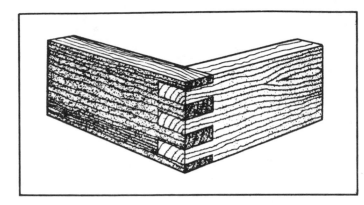

Fig. 2-63. Box corner joint.

general drawing you can design your own cabinets too. You may need special equipment for some of the joints illustrated here. Some ingenuity and time can often bring you good results with your own tools, however.

GOING TOGETHER

In this chapter you've learned about tools and techniques needed for building your own fitness center. You've considered the selection and use of common hand tools, power tools, and fasteners. Then you've seen an overall view of how homes are constructed and remodeled. Finally, you've taken a quick look at woodworking, especially joining. Additional information on tools and techniques will be

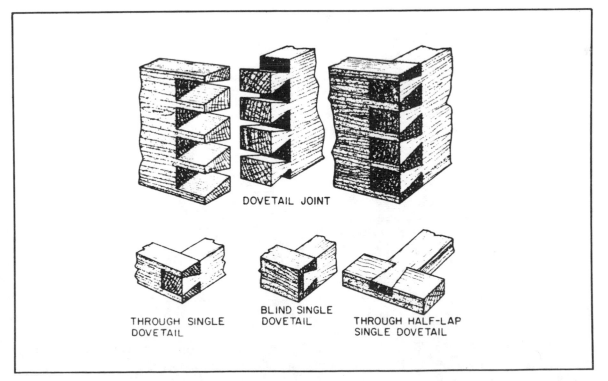

DOVETAIL JOINT

THROUGH SINGLE DOVETAIL

BLIND SINGLE DOVETAIL

THROUGH HALF-LAP SINGLE DOVETAIL

Fig. 2-64. Dovetail joints.

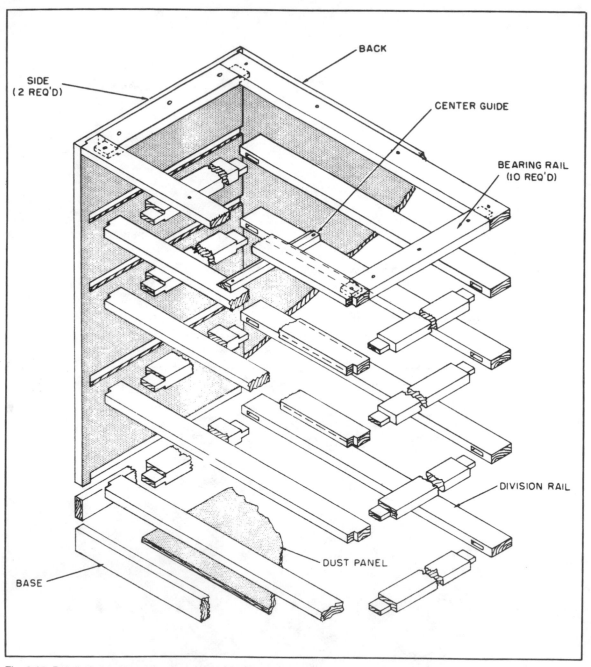

Fig. 2-65. Details for making a fitness equipment storage cabinet.

offered in the coming chapters on specific projects as they are needed. By gaining this knowledge of tools and techniques you can plan and build just about any type of fitness equipment you see or dream up.

Have fun!

3

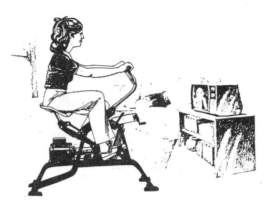

Exercise Room

T O LOOK YOUR BEST, TO FEEL YOUR BEST, AND to be able to do your best, you must exercise regularly (Fig. 3-1). That is human nature, and modern technology can't change it. When the activity required of you by your job and other duties falls below the level necessary to support good health, you must supplement it with planned activity. Your sense of well-being, your ability to perform, and even your survival depends on it.

You already know that regular, vigorous exercise increases muscle strength and endurance. It also improves the functioning of the lungs, heart, and blood vessels; promotes flexibility of the joints; releases mental and physical tensions; and aids in weight control or reduction. Medical research demonstrates that active persons have fewer heart attacks than sedentary persons. If they do suffer attacks, they recover more readily. More than half of all lower back pain is due to poor tone

and flexibility of the back and abdominal muscles. In many cases, this problem could be prevented or corrected by proper exercise. In short, exercise can make the difference. The options are mere existence or a full life.

This chapter will guide you in making that difference easier to enjoy. In the first part you'll learn how to plan and build an exercise room or area in your home. In the second part you'll find out how to build some useful exercise equipment—plus how to use your room with no equipment at all.

Let's get started.

YOUR EXERCISE ROOM

Finding a place to exercise on a regular basis is often a problem and can be a stumbling block to the beginning of a worthwhile exercise program. Let's move that stumbling block right now by finding a good place for regular exercise.

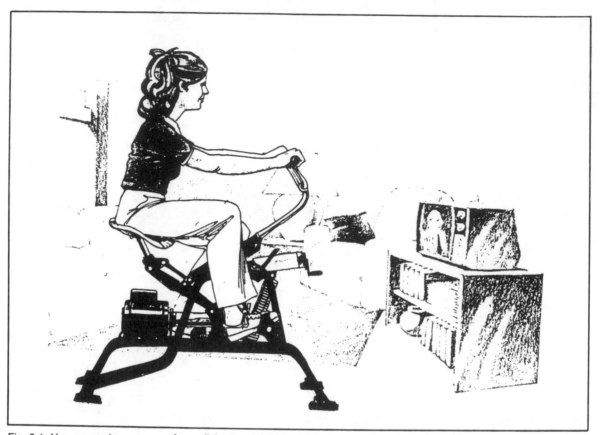

Fig. 3-1. You can make a corner of your living room into an exercise room. (Courtesy Exercycle)

Your exercise room may actually be part of an existing room in your home or apartment. If your exercise program includes jumping rope, aerobics, or a round trampoline needing only a few square feet of space, you may be able to store equipment in a closet or under a bed. Whatever space you can find, make sure it is adequate and available when you need it. Don't make plans to use part of your bedroom at 5 A.M. if your partner regularly sleeps until 6:30.

Once you've established your exercise program and found an adequate exercise "room" that's available when you need it, you can experiment to discover what you want in your ultimate exercise room. It may be nothing more than what you have; or it may be a com-

plete gym and fitness bath with access to an outdoor fitness center. The choices are yours.

You'll probably soon outgrow your pullout exercise "room" or area and want to expand into a regular location where you can store and use your growing inventory of exercise equipment. For so many homes with already limited space this means moving to the basement.

REMODELING THE BASEMENT

Many houses are now designed so that one or more rooms on the lower floors are constructed on a concrete slab. In multilevel houses, this area may include a family room, a spare bedroom, or a study. Furthermore, it is sometimes necessary to provide a room for recreation or exercise in the basement of an existing house. Thus, in a new house or in remodeling the basement of an existing one, several factors should be considered, including insulation, waterproofing, and vapor resistance. In the coming pages you'll learn how to make basement rooms into exercise rooms by working with floors, walls, and ceilings.

BASEMENT FLOORS

In remodeling a basement room into an exercise room, provision should be made to reduce heat loss and prevent ground moisture movement. Perimeter insulation reduces heat loss, and a vapor barrier under the slab prevents problems caused by a concrete floor damp from ground moisture (Figs. 3-2 and 3-3). Providing these essential details, however, is somewhat more difficult in existing construction than in new construction.

The installation of a vapor barrier over an existing, unprotected concrete slab is normally required when the floor is at or below the outside ground level and some type of finish floor is used. Flooring manufacturers often recommend that preparation of the slab for wood strip flooring consist of the following steps:

Step 1. Mop or spread a coating of tar or asphalt mastic followed by an asphalt felt paper.

Step 2. Lay short lengths of 2-by-4-inch screeds in a coating of tar or asphalt, spacing the rows about 12 inches apart, starting at one wall and ending at the opposite wall.

Step 3. Place insulation around the perimeter, between screeds, where the outside ground level is near the basement floor elevation.

Step 4. Install wood strip flooring across the wood screeds.

This system can be varied somewhat by placing a conventional vapor barrier of good quality directly over the slab. Two-by-four-inch furring strips spaced 12 to 16 inches apart are then anchored to the slab with concrete nails or with other types of commercial anchors. Some leveling of the 2 × 4s might be

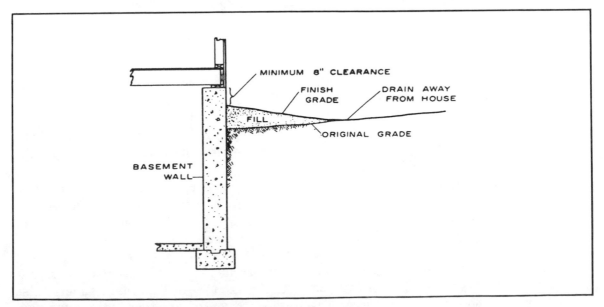

Fig. 3-2. Sloping the finish grade for drainage away from your basement.

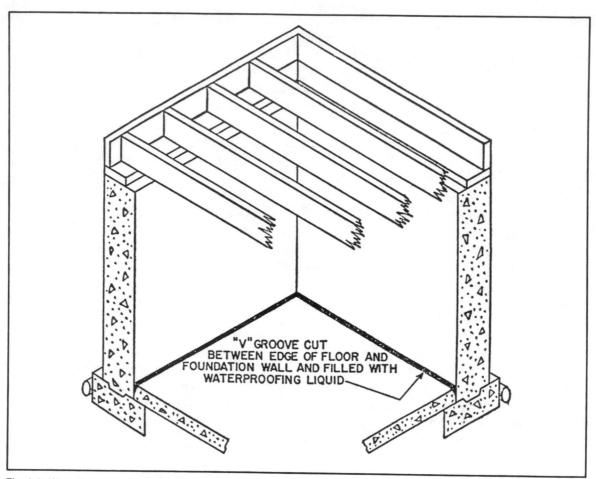

Fig. 3-3. Watertight seam on basement wall and floor.

required. Strip flooring is then nailed to the furring strips after perimeter insulation is placed (Fig. 3-4). If a wood block flooring is desired, a plywood subflooring may be used over the furring strips. Plywood, ½ or ⅝ inch thick, is normally used if the edges are un-blocked and furring strips are spaced 16 inches or more apart.

When insulation is not required around the perimeter because of the height of the outside grade above the basement floor, a much simpler method can be used for wood block or other type of tile finish. An asphalt mastic coating, followed by a good vapor bar-

rier, serves as a base for the tile. An adhesive recommended by the flooring manufacturer is then used over the vapor barrier, after which the wood tile is applied. It is important that a smooth, vapor-tight base be provided for the tile.

Such floor construction should be used only when drain tile is placed at the outside footings and soil conditions are favorable. When the slab or walls of an existing house incline to be damp, it is often difficult to ensure a dry basement. Under such conditions, it is often best to use resilient tile or similar finish over some type of stable base such as plywood.

This construction is preceded by insulation of vapor barriers and protective coatings.

BASEMENT WALLS

Using an interior finish over masonry basement walls will make your exercise room more enjoyable. Furthermore, if the outside wall is partially exposed, it's a good idea to use insulation between the wall and the inside finish. Waterproofing the wall is important if there is any possibility of moisture entry. It can be done by applying one of the many waterproof coatings available to the inner surface of the masonry (Figs. 3-5 and 3-6).

After the wall has been waterproofed, furring strips are normally used to prepare the wall for interior finish. A 2-by-2-inch bottom plate is anchored to the floor at the junction of the wall and floor. A 2-by-2-inch or larger top plate is fastened to the bottom of the joists, to joist blocks, or anchored to the wall (Fig. 3-7).

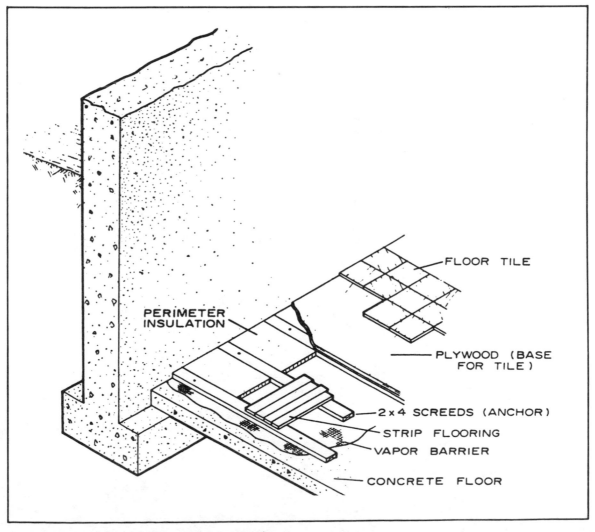

FLOOR TILE

PLYWOOD (BASE FOR TILE)

PERIMETER INSULATION

2 x 4 SCREEDS (ANCHOR)

STRIP FLOORING

VAPOR BARRIER

CONCRETE FLOOR

Fig. 3-4. Basement floor details for existing construction.

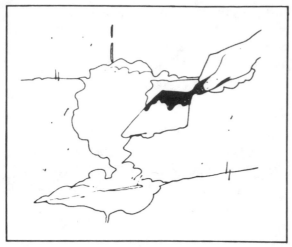

Fig. 3-5. Sealing basement walls.

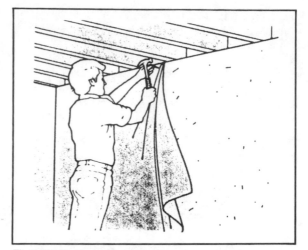

Fig. 3-6. Installing a plastic vapor barrier to reduce basement condensation. (Courtesy Georgia-Pacific)

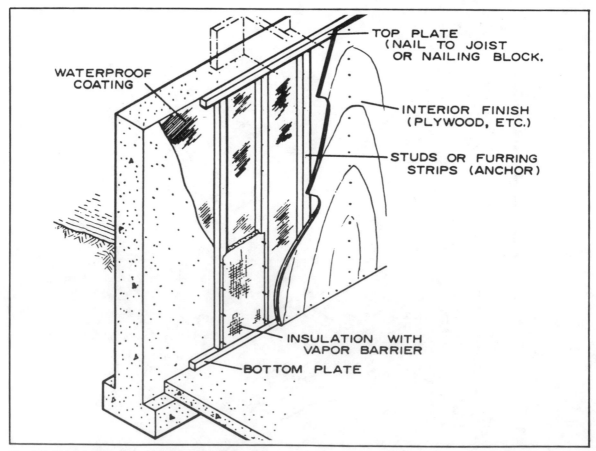

Fig. 3-7. Using furring strips to finish a basement wall.

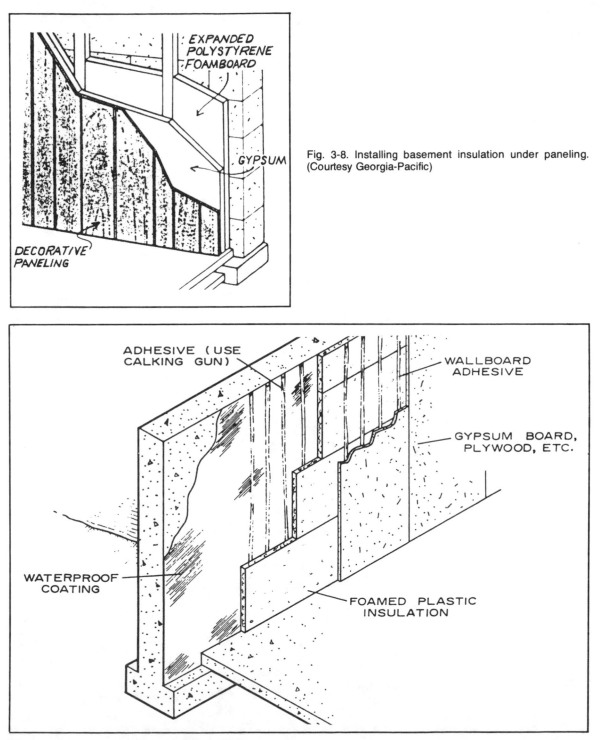

Fig. 3-8. Installing basement insulation under paneling. (Courtesy Georgia-Pacific)

EXPANDED POLYSTYRENE FOAMBOARD

GYPSUM

DECORATIVE PANELING

ADHESIVE (USE CALKING GUN)

WALLBOARD ADHESIVE

GYPSUM BOARD, PLYWOOD, ETC.

WATERPROOF COATING

FOAMED PLASTIC INSULATION

Fig. 3-9. Basement wall finish without furring strips.

Studs or furring strips, 2 by 2 inches or larger, are then placed between top and bottom plates, anchoring them at the center when necessary with concrete nails or similar fasteners. Electrical outlets and conduit should be installed and insulation with vapor barrier placed between the furring strips. The interior finish of gypsum board, fiberboard, plywood, or other material is then installed (Fig. 3-8). Furring strips are commonly spaced 16 inches on center, but this depends on the type of thickness of the interior finish.

Foamed plastic insulation is sometimes used on masonry walls without furring. It is important that the inner face of the wall be smooth and level without protrusions when this method is used. After the wall has been waterproofed, ribbons of adhesive are applied to the walls and sheets of foam insulation installed (Fig. 3-9). Drywall adhesive is then applied and the gypsum board, plywood, or other finish pressed in place. Most foam-plastic insulations have some vapor resistance in themselves, so the need for a separate barrier is not as great as when blanket-type insulation is used. Figure 3-10 shows exterior basement drainage.

BASEMENT CEILINGS

Some type of finish is usually desirable for the ceiling of your basement exercise room. Gypsum board, plywood, or fiberboard sheets may be used and nailed directly to the joints. Acoustic ceiling tile and similar materials

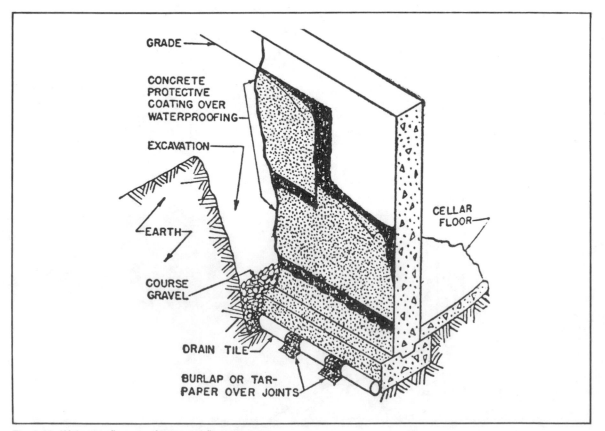

Fig. 3-10. Waterproofing your basement fitness center.

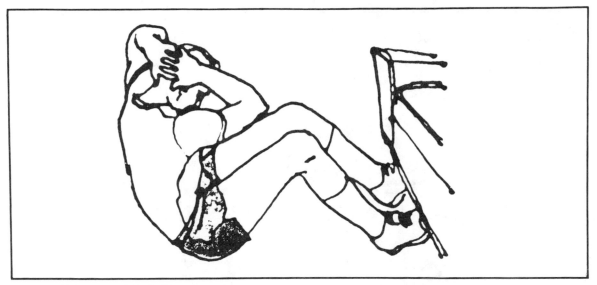

Fig. 3-11. Using a couch to do fitness exercises.

normally require additional nailing areas. This may be supplied by 1-by-2-inch or 1-by-3-inch strips nailed across the joists and spaced to conform to the size of the ceiling tile.

A suspended ceiling may also be used. This can consist of a system of light metal angles hung from the ceiling joists. Tiles are then dropped in place. This will also aid in decreasing sound transfer from the rows above. Remember to install ceiling lights, heat supply and return ducts, or other utilities before the finish is applied.

FROM BASEMENT TO EXERCISE ROOM

Finishing off your basement for use as an exercise room is just one way of finding space for your fitness center. Others have been covered in the first two chapters and will be offered in coming pages. The important thing is that a regular place be found or developed that offers both the space and the commitment for better health.

The simplest fitness or exercise equipment to find and use are the objects already around your home, such as furniture (Fig. 3-11), chairs (Figs. 3-12 through 3-14) and closet bars (Fig. 3-15). You don't have to have a special area for these simple exercise aids.

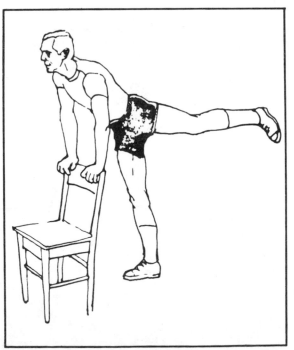

Fig. 3-12. Using a dining room chair for the back leg swing.

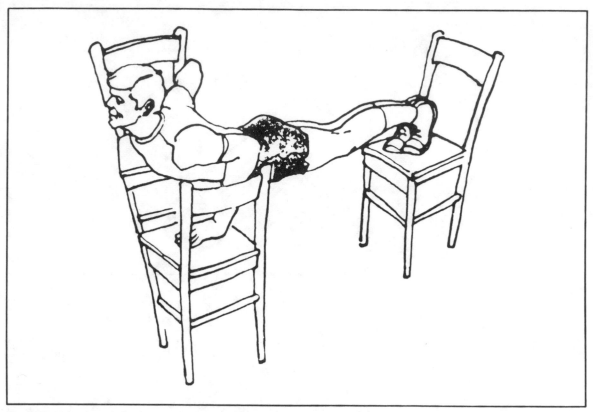

Fig. 3-13. Using two chairs for an advanced version of the push-up.

Fig. 3-14. Using a dining room chair for sitting leg raises.

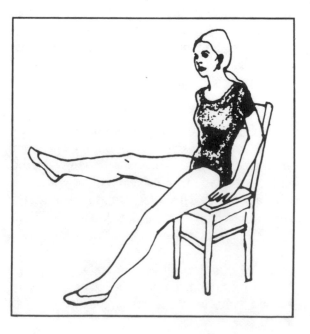

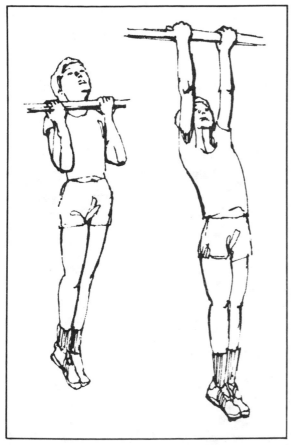

Fig. 3-15. Youngsters can use a sturdy clothes bar in a closet for chin-ups.

You will probably soon outgrow basic components such as these, however, and decide to buy, install, or build your own exercise equipment.

EXERCISE BICYCLES

There are three areas to consider in your plan for exercise and exercise equipment: cardiovascular, strength, and flexibility. Many people feel a need to develop their heart for remedial or preventative reasons. One of the most popular exercise equipment units for this is the stationary bicycle (Figs. 3-16 through 3-21). Some are truly stationary—offering only leg movement similar to jogging. More

elaborate ergometers are complete physical fitness machines that offer a variety of exercise possibilities, such as swimming, rowing, stretching, and even chin-ups.

Of course, purchasing an exercise or stationary bicycle should be a careful study of what's available and what's in your budget. A simple stationary bicycle can cost as little as $80 on sale; but a more complete exercise bicycle can approach $500.

Setting up your stationary bicycle is simple enough. Unpack it from the carton (save the box for a couple of weeks), check the shipping list and make sure that all parts are included. Loose parts often include the seat assembly, handlebar assembly, pedals, and tools. You may first have to remove a wooden frame before assembling your bike. Once everything's checked over, you can insert and adjust the handlebar assembly and install the seat and the pedals. On most exercise bikes, the left pedal (as you would sit on the bike) is marked with an "L" while the right pedal has an "R" stamped on the end. The opposite threads of these two pedals help insure that normal action tightens rather than loosens them.

If you have an electric exercise bike, remember to make sure you've placed your bike near an outlet—no extension cords if at all possible. Also make sure that you've read all the instructions before plugging the unit in.

If you want, you can also purchase or build a simple rack that will allow you to turn your regular bicycle into an exercise bicycle.

ROWING MACHINES

Another popular exercise unit for developing cardiovascular strength is the rowing machine (Figs. 3-22 through 3-24). They are more costly than a basic stationary bike but not as much as a powered exercise bicycle. Their greatest advantage beyond exercise is their portability. Rowing machines can be shoved under the bed, stood up in a closet, or placed in the car trunk for vacations and travel.

In shopping for a rowing machine, look for one that is built to stand up to use; that is, make sure that the tubing and joints are solid and will not be excessively stressed as you grow in strength. Also, make sure you check the handles. A comfortable grip is important to minimize blisters and sore hands. As with any piece of equipment, purchase one that you've tried out for more than a couple moments. No salesperson minds having someone spending ten minutes to an hour using a demonstrator in

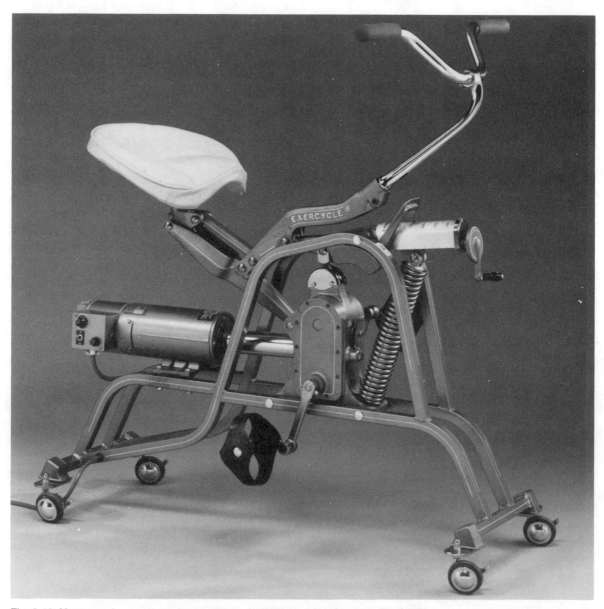

Fig. 3-16. Your exercise room can begin with an exercise bicycle. (Courtesy Exercycle)

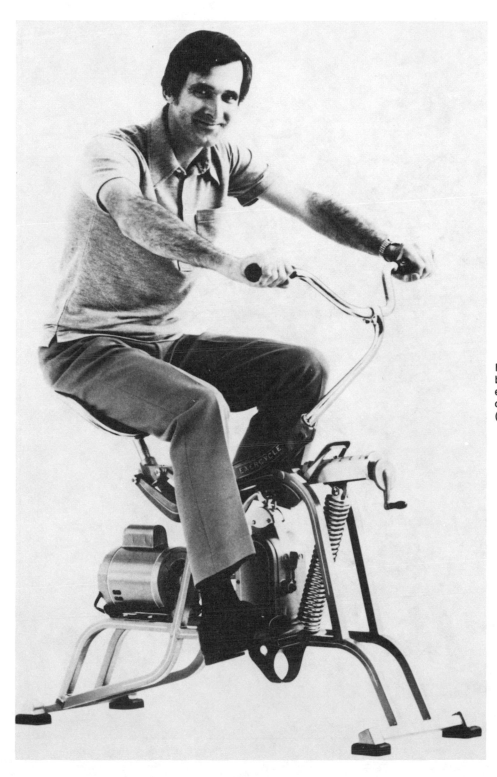

Fig. 3-17. An exercise bicycle offers serious exercise after a long day at the office. (Courtesy Exercycle)

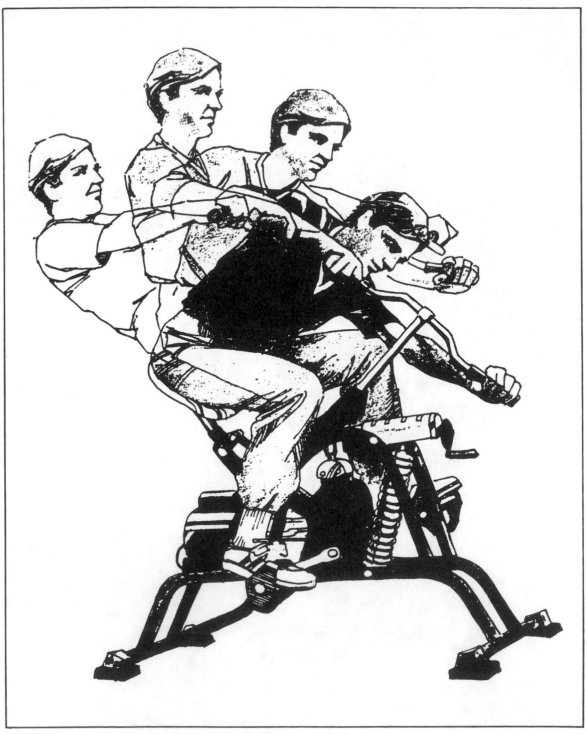

Fig. 3-18. Exercise bicycle movements. (Courtesy Exercycle)

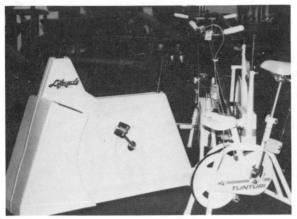

Fig. 3-19. Two types of stationary bikes.

the store as it often helps sell more units.

TREADMILLS

Many regular exercisers feel that the treadmill

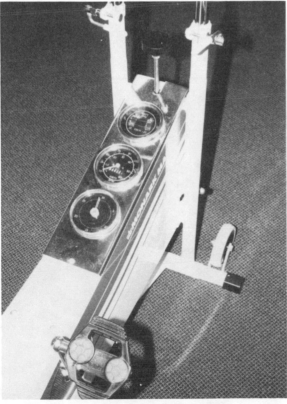

Fig. 3-20. Exercise bikes offer metering options.

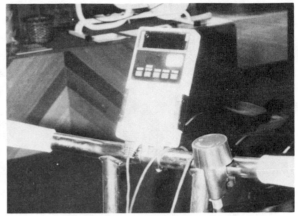

Fig. 3-21. Pulse meter mounted on an exercise bike.

is one of the best indoor exercise units you can buy. It allows you to walk or even jog in all types of climates, weather conditions, and neighborhoods. You will probably use a treadmill more often than you would jog (Figs. 3-25 and 3-26).

If your skills or budget dictate, you can build your own treadmill with simple tools. Build a wooden frame surrounding fifteen to twenty ⅜-inch-by-24-inch rods covered by a heavy-duty, cotton-backed, vinyl treadmill belt.

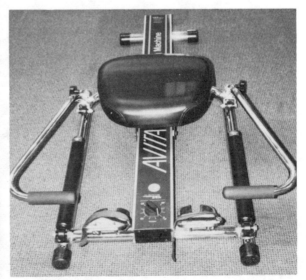

Fig. 3-22. Rowing machine.

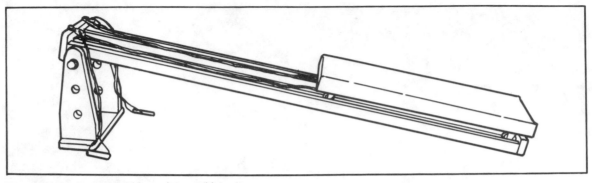

Fig. 3-23. You can make this rowing machine.

KNEELING BENCH

One of the easiest exercise aids to build is the kneeling bench. Kneeling benches can be used for a variety of exercises including push-ups, lift-ups, and working with weights. Follow the plans in Figs. 3-27 and 3-28. Cut the parts to size, make the dado cuts or grooves for the legs, then attach the legs and edging with glue and dowels or screws. Sand the bench and finish as desired.

OTHER EXERCISE EQUIPMENT

There are numerous other pieces of exercise equipment that you can buy or build for your exercise room, including exercise pads (Fig. 3-29), rebounders or minitrampolines (Fig. 3-30), antigravity racks (Figs. 3-31 and 3-32), and many others. The limitations of your exercise room are those you impose: economics and motivation. You'll find a wide variety of equipment to fit your exercise needs.

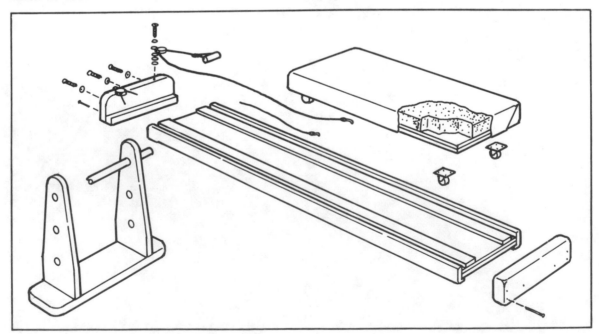

Fig. 3-24. Construction details for your rowing machine.

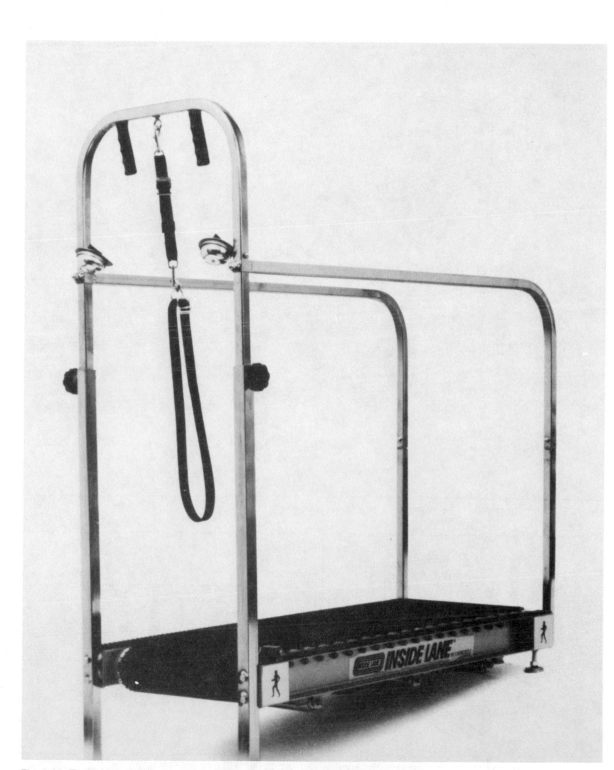

Fig. 3-25. Typical treadmill you can buy for your exercise room. (Courtesy Exercycle)

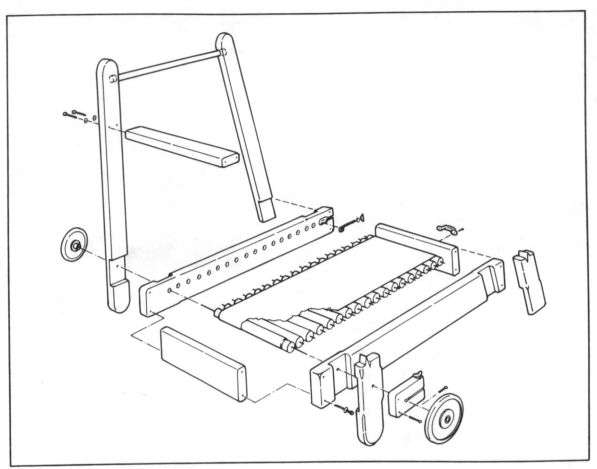

Fig. 3-26. Construction details for making your own portable treadmill.

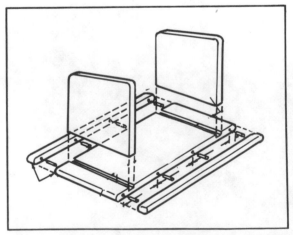

Fig. 3-27. Construction details for making your own kneeling bench.

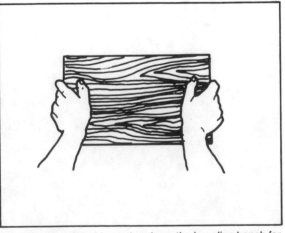

Fig. 3-28. How to hold your hands on the kneeling bench for advanced push-ups.

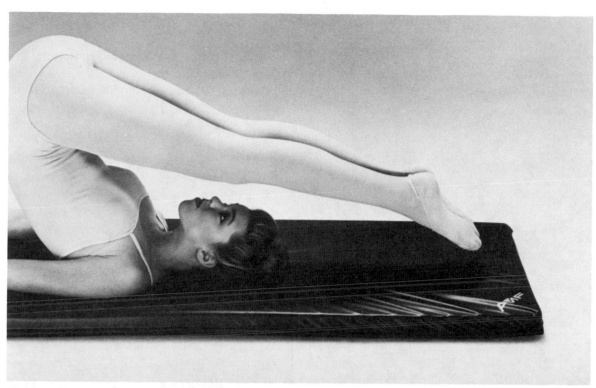

Fig. 3-29. Floor exercise mat. (Courtesy AMF)

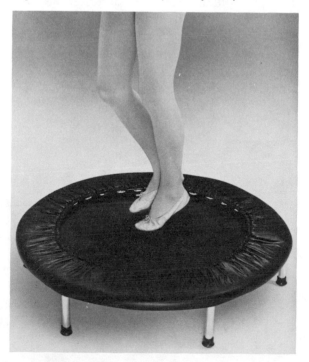

Fig. 3-30. Rebound exerciser. (Courtesy AMF)

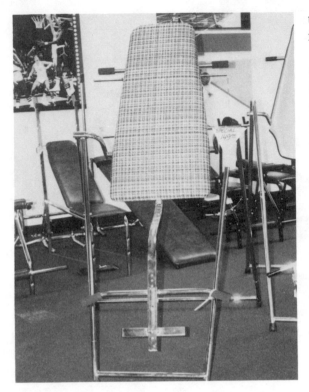

Fig. 3-31. Antigravity bench.

RULES FOR CONDUCTING EXERCISE

Exercise is work, but it can also be fun. To make it more fun than work, follow these rules for efficient and safe exercise.

Rule 1—Warm-up Rule. Take it easy and at least do some preliminary bending, stretching, and running in place before you get into more serious exercises. Warm-up is protective against injuries and the sudden development of an oxygen deficiency.

Rule 2—Regulate Your Dosage. Build up the intensity of the work gradually, push up to a peak of effort, then taper off.

Rule 3—Work Out Progessively. Improvement depends upon a gradual increase in the total amount of work done. The progression is equivalent to 100, 300, 500 calories of heat, corresponding to 30 minutes, 45 min-

utes, an hour of work with gradual increase in intensity.

Rule 4—Recuperation. Keep moving; don't sit down. Breathe as deeply as possible and force the breath out explosively. Stretch any muscles which have been worked hard. Avoid smoking which constricts lung capillaries.

Rule 5—Work Various Parts. Neck, shoulders, chest, upper back, waist, lower back, abdomen, legs, and feet. In addition, there should be some running (perhaps in place) or rowing, skating, swimming, cycling, skiing—some continuous rhythmical work for endurance, forcing the circulation and respiration.

Rule 6—For Heart Protection. Warm up gradually before exposure to hard work or extreme cold or heat.

Rule 7—Circulation. Circulation is usually better in the lying rather than the sitting or standing position. It is better in a cool environment than a hot environment. Rhythmic movement is the greatest boost to circulation, but tense (static) efforts may block the circulation more or less. Forced breathing helps the circulation along with walking, running, swimming, skating, skiing, dancing, rowing, and rhythmic calisthenics.

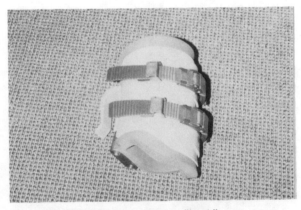

Fig. 3-32. Antigravity leg support or "boot."

Rule 8—Workout Time. Best for most people is about three to four hours after meals; but people who sit nearly all day need to get up and move about at least every hour. Many work out before breakfast, during their lunch hour, or between 9:00 and 10:00 at night. One can adapt to any reasonable schedule. The main caution is to avoid hard work right after meals.

Rule 9—Take Cool Baths. Normally baths should be hot (short), then cool (long) as cool baths are recuperative, help the circulation, and stir up the metabolism more than hot baths. However, a hot bath is all right just before bed.

Rule 10—Using fuel. Exercise will burn up from 1 to 15 calories per minute, depending upon the intensity of the exercise. So the length of time you exercise at a given rate determines how much fuel is used. To burn one pound of fat requires 4320 to 4380 calories, according to the respiratory efficiency. To burn fat reserves takes time. There is no short cut.

In addition to the above ten rules, here are a few more dos and don'ts for exercising.

Exercise mildly or moderately a minimum of three times a week. There should be a minimum of a 15-minute aerobic or calisthenic segment in each exercise session.

Breathe freely when exercising. Do not hold your breath.

Arm support or hanging exercises may increase your blood pressure. This is particularly true for older persons. If you are older, do this type of exercise with caution. These are not recommended for persons with hypertension and/or other medical problems.

Avoid back hyperextension if you have lower back problems. Back hyperextensions include lying on the stomach and lifting both legs and both arms at the same time or bending backward in an upright position. If you do perform back hyperextension exercises, follow them with trunk flexion.

Isometric exercises develop strength only in the position performed. This type of exercise may be dangerous for those with cardiovascular problems because it prevents blood flow and circulation momentarily. If you do perform this exercise, don't hold your breath.

Avoid freely swinging the body against a fixed joint. Heels need to come up when twisting, knees should always be slightly flexed when bending forward.

Do bent-knee sit-ups. They tone the abdominal muscles and will not strain the lower back when done properly.

Double leg lifts are discouraged unless the small of the back can be maintained flat against the floor at all times during the exercise.

All stretching should be done slowly. Bouncing exercises may cause lower back discomfort and could also cause muscle soreness and straining.

When on your back, keep one or both knees flexed with the foot or feet on the floor. This will avoid lower back strain.

Try not to do more than two consecutive exercises for one particular muscle group. Using muscle groups antagonistically is more comfortable. It will help to avoid local fatigue. Do one set of sit-ups, then an exercise which relaxes or uses that muscle group in another way, and then a second set of sit-ups.

There should be no pain involved in exercise. Avoid straining and pushing yourself to the extent that you are exhausted.

Remember to exercise sensibly. Train, don't strain. Follow the guidelines.

WORKING OUT

Whether you've set aside an area to drag out your jump rope and exercise mat, or you've remodeled the basement for your ergocycle, treadmill, and other equipment, your exercise "room" can offer you both fitness and fun.

Next, we'll consider how to build your own weight room for developing strength and body tone.

4

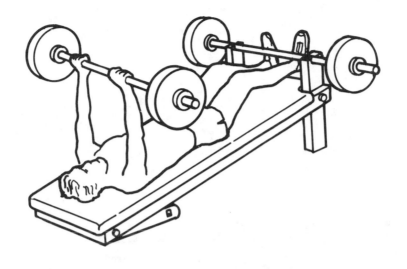

Weight Room

WEIGHT TRAINING IS A SYSTEMATIC SERIES of resistance exercises designed to promote physical development and conditioning. It's also effective for rehabilitating persons who have suffered injury or illness. In this chapter you'll learn how to plan, install, and use your own weight room at home (Fig. 4-1).

First, let's define some terms for those who are interested in weight training but who haven't entered the field yet. *Strength* is the ability to exert force or overcome resistance. It is an important component in sports performance and many forms of physical work. *Power*, as used here, refers to a combination of strength and speed. It is the ability to apply strength in an "explosive" movement. *Muscle endurance* is the ability of the muscles to continue to contract—to do work—over long periods.

Weight training, when performed properly, may contribute to *flexibility*: the ability of the joints to move through a full range of motion. Flexibility is enhanced when opposing muscles are in balance and the muscles and connective tissue are of proper length and elasticity.

Training with weights, under certain conditions, may also contribute to another major component of physical fitness—*circulatory endurance* or the efficiency of the cardiovascular and respiratory systems. Such conditions require that exercises be done rhythmically and consecutively with only short rests (30 seconds or less) in between exercise bouts. Otherwise, minimal circulatory improvement will be gained.

Because of it's effectiveness and the fact that rather precise routines of progressively increased resistance can be set up, the use of weight training is increasing rapidly in athletic conditioning and skill training, school and college physical education, public fitness pro-

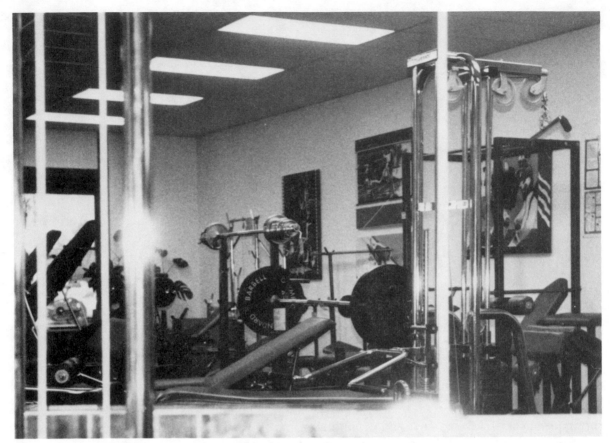

Fig. 4-1. You can select from many types of weight room equipment at your local fitness shop.

grams, rehabilitation programs, and individual conditioning regimens. This last group is the one that seems to be growing most dramatically and has the greatest need of home weight rooms.

WEIGHT TRAINING

A well-chosen sequence of weight exercises, pursued regularly over a period of time, can bring about significant improvement in the fitness components just discussed. Physical condition, posture, and appearance can be improved, body measurements reapportioned, and sagging body contours firmed up. Weight training is particularly worthwhile in helping the physically undeveloped person because the

regimen and goals can be easily adapted to individual needs and capacities. Progress is obvious in a relatively short time and is satisfying and stimulating to further effort. Important psychological benefits in poise, self-discipline, self-direction, and self-realization are often derived. Significant improvement in sports performance can be obtained through selected exercises as well as through those that build overall strength, flexibility, power, and endurance.

Although most weight training programs are for men and boys, women and girls can benefit too. Progressive resistance exercises can be easily adapted to each girl's capacity, ability, and needs. Most American girls lack adequate strength in arms, shoulders, and trunk and could profit from a developmental routine.

Before considering weight training equipment, let's review some of the general principles of weight training. They can help you decide whether weight training is for you as well as what type of equipment to select.

Studies have found that training with submaximal loads of as low as two-thirds or more of maximum strength twice weekly and maximal loads once weekly will result in as much strength improvement as training maximally three times weekly. The load with which to train for optimum improvement in strength, when training three times weekly for one set each, lies between 3RM (three repetitions of lifting the maximum weight) to 9RM.

Training with the 2RM for six sets, three times weekly, is as effective for increasing strength as training with the 6RM for three sets, three times weekly. Training with the 6RM for three sets, three times weekly, is more effective for increasing strength than training with either the 2RM or 10RM for three sets, three times weekly.

Training once weekly with the 10RM for one set will increase strength significantly after the first week of training and each week up to at least the sixth week. Weight training with the 10RM for three sets, twice weekly, is just as effective for increasing strength as training the same way three times weekly.

No particular sequence of performance in training with different proportions of 10RM maximum strength will be more effective than any other sequence for strength improvement as long as one set of 10RM is performed each training session. Three sets for each lift are more effective for increasing strength than training for one or two sets.

The number of training days per week for optimum improvement in strength is not known. Significant increases have occurred training one day weekly to five days per week for beginners, but in these instances only one lift was performed.

Training with several lifts, four or five days per week, may not be as effective for increasing strength as training the same way two or three times per week. The greater muscular fatigue experienced from training more frequently may prevent sufficient recuperation between training sessions and, therefore, reduce the rate of progression.

A program of three training sessions per week, provided the number of different lifts is not excessive, should not be too few for excellent results. A beginner should start with eight to ten lifts and then add or reduce this number according to his or her recuperative ability. A fourth workout per week may be added later when the individual attains improved physical conditions.

SELECTING WEIGHTS

As mentioned earlier, weight training is a systematic series of resistance exercises designed to promote physical development and conditioning. This resistance is developed against weighted equipment or *weights*. The two most common types of weights are dumbbells and barbells. *Dumbbells* (Fig. 4-2) are smaller, fixed weights usually held in each hand to offer resistance in a number of exercises. They are easily used and stored and require little space. *Barbells* are larger, adjustable weights including the bar (Fig. 4-3) and assorted weights (Fig. 4-4) that can be equally added to the ends of the bar for resistance.

In addition, there are numerous types and sizes of fitness machines (Figs. 4-5 through 4-9) that offer adjustable resistance to movement. They have become increasingly popular with people who desire compact weight train-

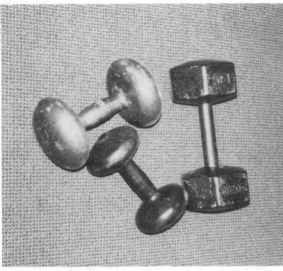

Fig. 4-2. Hand dumbbells.

ing systems for the home. You can also make your own weight training equipment simply and easily by using pipes set in concrete that has been poured into coffee cans or other containers, springs and pulleys, or other apparatus.

USING WEIGHTS

Here are descriptions of the more common weight training exercises. Consider each of them for your own needs and to help you in selecting equipment (Fig. 4-10) for your weight room.

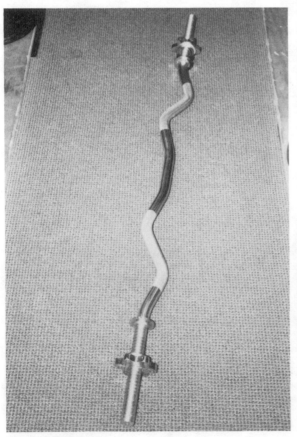

Fig. 4-3. Barbell bar.

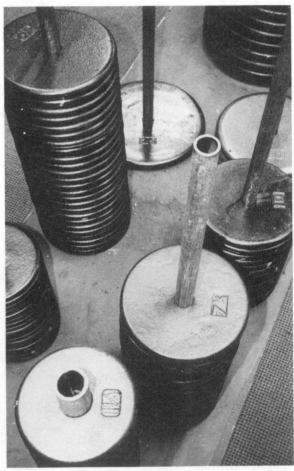

Fig. 4-4. Barbell weights.

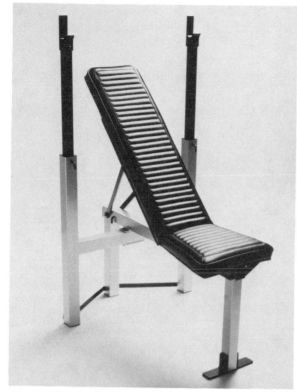

Fig. 4-5. Weight bench.

higher than shoulders. Then lower the bar to the starting position. Only shoulders and arms should move during this exercise. Inhale when raising weight and exhale when lowering it.

Side Bends

To start, stand erect with your feet spread comfortably apart, about 10 to 12 inches and knees slightly flexed. Place arms at sides, each hand holding a dumbbell, knuckles out. Bend torso to the right as far as possible, keeping dumbbells near the body. Avoid leaning forward or backward and keep both feet flat on the floor. Then return to the starting position. Next, bend to the left and return to the starting position.

Half Squats

To begin, stand erect with feet comfortably

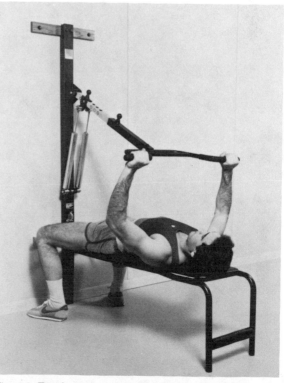

Fig. 4-6. Tension-type weight bench. (Courtesy AMF)

Military Press

To start, stand erect with feet comfortably apart and chest high. With hands shoulder-width apart, grasp the barbell with palms facing legs and raise the bar to the upper chest (palms now facing forward). Then press the bar upward overhead until the elbows are fully extended. Finally, lower the bar to the chest position. Remember to inhale when raising the weight and exhale when lowering it. This exercise may also be performed from the starting position with the bar behind the neck.

Upright Rowing

To start, stand erect with feet comfortably apart and hold bar in front of thighs, hands about 6 inches apart with palms facing legs. Pull the bar up to the chin, bringing elbows apart, heels on a 2-by-4-foot board. Rest barbells across the shoulders behind neck, hands grasping bar with palms facing away from body. Then lower your body until knee joint is approximately at right angle. Finally, straighten legs to the erect position. The heels should be kept in contact with the board when performing this exercise. Also, keep your head up and back straight. Exhale when squatting, straighten up from heels, and inhale when rising to erect position.

Bench Press

To start, lie flat on your back on the bench with legs bent and astride, feet on the floor. Grasp the bar with hands more than shoulder-width

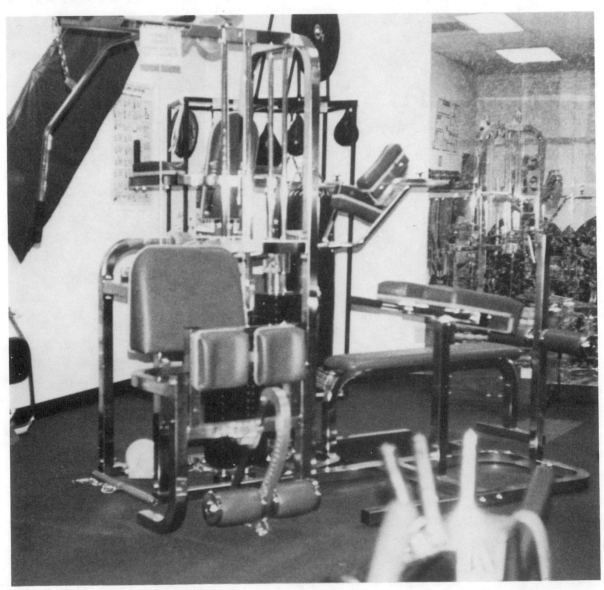

Fig. 4-7. Numerous types of weight equipment.

extended downward with the bar resting lightly against the front of your thighs. Count 1: flex elbows fully, lifting the bar upward toward your chest. Keep elbows close to your sides and avoid raising your shoulders. Don't lean backward or "bounce" the bar with a leg motion. Count 2: return to the starting position. Inhale on count 1 and exhale on count 2.

Sit-Ups

To begin, lie on back with legs extended and feet about 12 inches apart. Hold a weight behind your neck. Ankles should be held or placed under a barrier to keep the heels in contact with the floor. First, curl up to a sitting position, carrying through far enough to touch

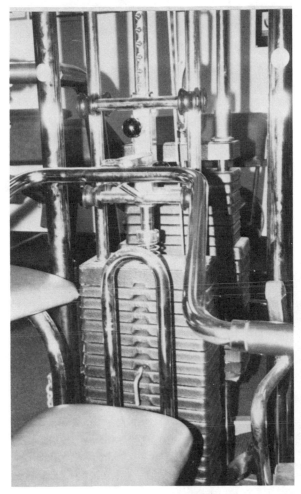

Fig. 4-8. Professional weight bench details.

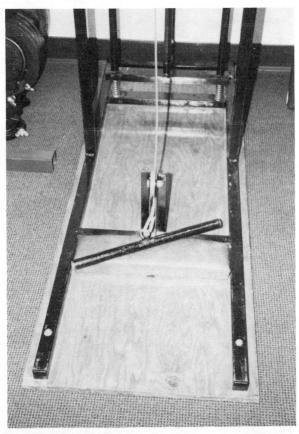

Fig. 4-9. Simple homemade weight lifting bar mounted on a platform for easy moving.

apart, palms away from your face, and arms extended. Lower the weights to your chest and exhale. Then raise the weights straight up while inhaling. It's a good idea to have someone assist you in getting the weights into position to lift and in taking the weights off the bench stand after the exercise is completed.

Curls

To start, stand erect with your feet spread comfortably apart, about 10 to 12 inches, and knees slightly flexed. Grasp the bar with hands shoulder-width apart, palms facing out, arms

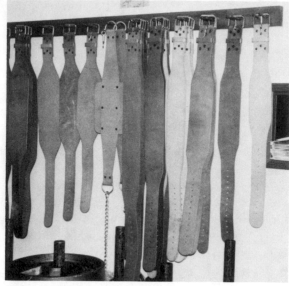
Fig. 4-10. Weight belts.

elbows to knees. The knees may be flexed slightly during this action. Then return to the starting position. This exercise should be smooth, curling up and down.

Backward Dumbbell Flings

To start, stand while bent forward at the waist with feet wide apart, (20 to 30 inches), knees slightly flexed, trunk straight and parallel to the ground, and head up looking forward.

Grasp a dumbbell in each hand, palms toward side of body, arms hanging vertically downward. Begin by flinging arms backward and sideward from shoulders, raising dumbbells in an arc as far as they will go keeping elbows extended. Hold the body stable and avoid raising the trunk or "bouncing" your legs. Then return the bells to the starting position. Remember to inhale during the fling and exhale as you return.

MAKE YOUR OWN BARBELLS

As you can see from the preceding description of popular weight training exercises, the barbell is one of the most useful pieces of equipment you can own. Many people purchase barbell sets at sporting good stores and large department stores. Others make their own (Figs. 4-11 through 4-13).

You can make a homemade set of barbells very easily. Begin with a bar made with a 1¼-inch steel rod or pipe approximately 5 feet 9 inches in length. To keep the weights in place, each end of the bar is made so that weight flanges slip into the slot on the bar. A collar is placed on the inside of each end of the bar, weights are added, and the end is capped with a second collar.

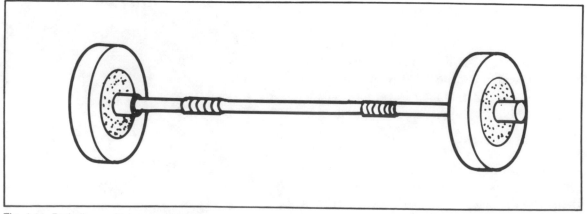
Fig. 4-11. Barbells you can make at home.

88

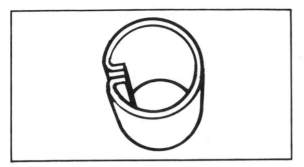

Fig. 4-12. Metal clasp you can make to attach weights to bar.

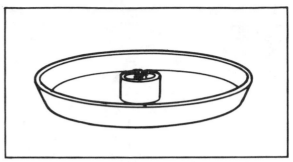

Fig. 4-13. Homemade barbell weight form with clasp.

The weights can be cast in coffee cans, cake pans, or even Frisbees, making sure that the weight flange is tall enough in the mold to go all the way through the weight. The weight is cast using premixed concrete, allowed to cure two to four days, and periodically dampened to minimize cracking. You can include chicken wire or other mesh to reinforce the weights. Finally, wrap the pipe with tape or rubber hose where your hands will grip.

MAKE YOUR OWN EXERCISE BENCH

Figures 4-14 and 4-15 illustrate how you can easily build your own exercise bench for weight lifting as well as numerous other excercises. The bench itself can be cut from ¾-inch or 1-inch interior grade plywood while the legs are constructed of 2 × 4s. Use screws rather than nails to fasten it together (see Chapter 2). Lock washers are also used to ensure strength and stability to your bench.

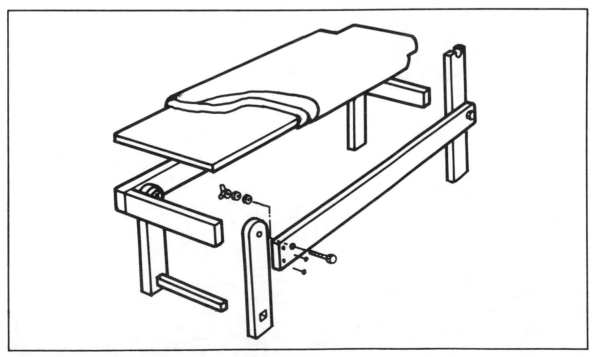

Fig. 4-14. Construction details for your own weight bench.

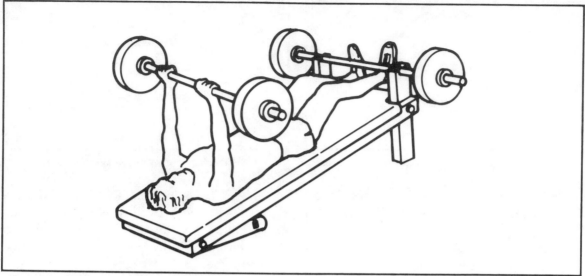

Fig. 4-15. Using your homemade weight bench.

MAKE YOUR OWN WALL WEIGHTS

By installing weights to a pulley attached to a wall you can make a wall weight set that will be both practical and inexpensive. The weights can be poured concrete, as are those used for the barbells, or they can be concrete blocks or bricks attached to the pull rope. The handle can be a short piece of pipe with the rope running through it and tied tight, or a U-shaped toilet tissue holder. It must be strong enough to withstand the resistance of the weights you use in your wall exercise unit.

PANELING YOUR WEIGHT ROOM

You might want to panel your weight room. The first step to paneling, once you've chosen the materials you need, is to locate the studs (Fig. 4-16). Studs are the vertical wood "skeleton" of most walls and are usually spaced 16 inches apart. This is what you will nail your paneling to.

Here's one quick method to try. Carefully remove the base and/or shoe molding and look for the heads of nails used to secure the drywall or plaster lath to the studs. If this method doesn't locate the studs for you, then start probing into the wall surface with a nail or small drill until you hit solid wood. Figure 4-17 illustrates how to probe. Furring strip installation is shown in Figs. 4-18 through 4-20.

Next, start in one corner of the room and measure floor-to-ceiling height for the first

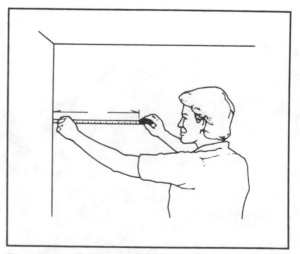

Fig. 4-16. The first step to installing paneling is locating the studs. (Courtesy Georgia-Pacific)

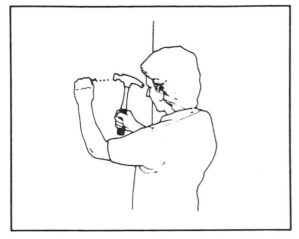

Fig. 4-17. Checking stud location. (Courtesy Georgia-Pacific)

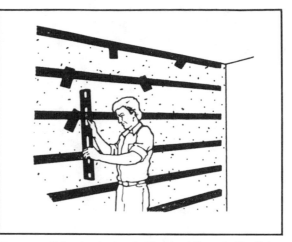

Fig. 4-19. Shimming for level. (Courtesy Georgia-Pacific)

panel. Subtract ½ inch to allow clearance top and bottom in order to maneuver the panel into place. Moldings will later cover this gap. Transfer your measurements to the first panel, using a pencil and straightedge for a clean line. All cutting should be done with a sharp saw with a minimum "set" (angling) to the teeth for reduced splintering. Use a crosscut handsaw with 10 or more teeth to the inch or a plywood blade in a table saw. If you use a portable circular saw or sabre saw, mark and cut panels from the back.

Cutouts for door and window sections, electrical switches, and outlets (Fig. 4-21) or heat registers require careful measurements. Take your dimensions from the edge of the last-applied panel for width and from the ceiling or floor for height. Transfer the measurements to the panel checking as you go. Unless you plan to add moldings around doors and windows, cutouts should fit snugly against the surrounding casing.

For electrical boxes, shut off the power and unscrew the protective plate to expose the

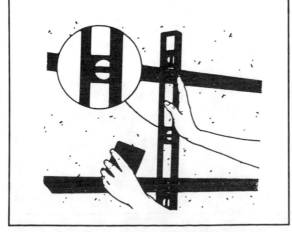

Fig. 4-18. Checking level. (Courtesy Georgia-Pacific)

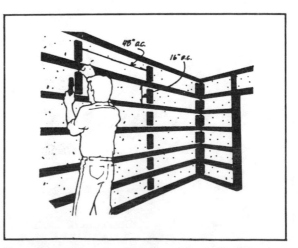

Fig. 4-20. Tacking strips. (Courtesy Georgia-Pacific)

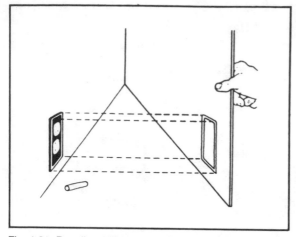

Fig. 4-21. Paneling utility cutout. (Courtesy Georgia-Pacific)

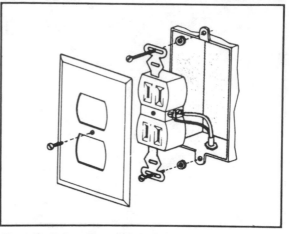

Fig. 4-23. Reinstalling utilities. (Courtesy Georgia-Pacific)

box. Then paint or run chalk around the box edges. Next, carefully position the panel and press it firmly over the box area, transferring the outline to the back of the panel. Drive small nails in each corner through the panel until they protrude through the face. Turn the panel over, drill two ¾-inch holes just inside the corners (Fig. 4-22) and use a keyhole or sabre saw to make the cutout. The hole can be up to ¼ inch oversize and still be covered when the protective switch plate is replaced (Fig. 4-23).

Installing Paneling

The first panel is the most important one, so take your time. Put the first panel in place (butted up against the corner of the room). Using the plumb bob (Fig. 4-24), make sure it's completely "plumb" or vertically true and that both left and right panel edges have wall studs directly behind them so they can be securely nailed in place. The "inside" edge should fit snugly into the corner of the room.

If the outer edge doesn't fit directly over a

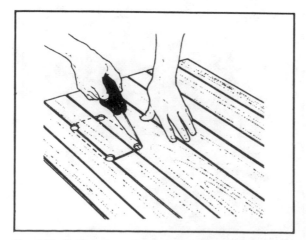

Fig. 4-22. Cutting the panel for the utility box. (Courtesy Georgia-Pacific)

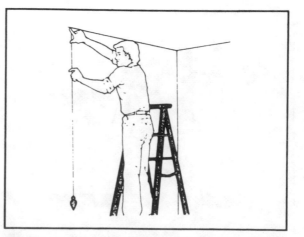

Fig. 4-24. Plumb lines can guide you in installing straight wall panels. (Courtesy Georgia-Pacific)

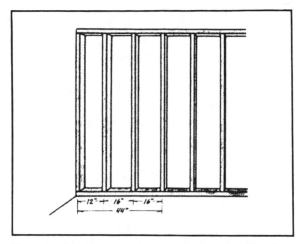

Fig. 4-25. Marking less-than-standard studs. (Courtesy Georgia-Pacific)

stud (Fig. 4-25), scribe or mark the panel on the inner edge (Fig. 4-26) and cut on the line. The outer edge should now come to the center of the stud—44 inches from the corner. This will provide room for nailing your next panel to the same stud. Okay so far? If not, look again at the measurement shown and visualize what would happen if you put a 48-inch panel against the 44-inch segment of wall.

Most paneling will have a groove every 16 inches so you can nail in the grooves—where

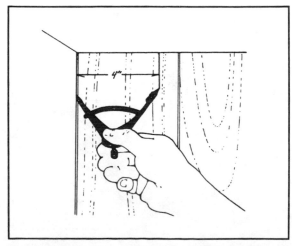

Fig. 4-26. Marking the cut. (Courtesy Georgia-Pacific)

nail holes are less visible—into the underlying studs. You can use regular small-headed finish nails (see Chapter 2) or colored paneling nails. For paneling directly to studs, use 3d (1¼-inch) nails. If you are nailing through any kind of wallboard or plaster, use 6d (2-inch) nails to get a solid bite into the stud. Space your nails 6 inches apart at the panel's edge and 12 inches apart in the panel field. Use your nail set to countersink the nailheads slightly below the surface, then fill with a matching putty stick. If you use colored panel nails, there's no need to countersink or use putty. Use 1-inch colored nails to secure paneling directly to studs or 1⅝-inch nails to apply paneling to wallboard or plaster.

The alternative method of using adhesive as your fastener eliminates the need for countersinking and hiding nailheads. You also won't have to line up panel edges and grooves directly over studs, if panels are applied over an existing wall surface. Adhesive may be applied directly to studs or over existing walls as long as the surface is sound and clean. Before you start, make certain that paneling is properly cut and fitted and that wall and panels are free of dirt and dust. Once the panel is applied with adhesive, adjustment is difficult. But the good news is that paneling applied with adhesive—if you do a careful job—has a more professional appearance!

A caulking gun with adhesive tube is the simplest method of application. Trim the tube to produce a ⅛-inch bead of adhesive. Apply a continuous bead of adhesive along the top, bottom, and side edges of the fitted panel you're about to put up (Fig. 4-27). On intermediate studs, apply beads of adhesive 3 inches long and 6 inches apart. With scrap plywood or panel used as a spacer at floor level, set the panel carefully in place and press firmly along edges and stud lines, spreading the underlying adhesive. To make the bond truly solid, use a

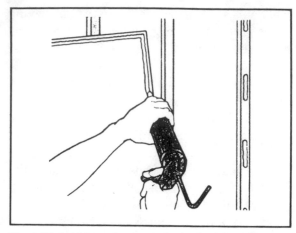

Fig. 4-27. Applying adhesive to the back of the wall panel. (Courtesy Georgia-Pacific)

rubber mallet or hammer and padded block to tap over the glue lines.

Make sure you read the adhesive manufacturer's instructions carefully. Some require the panel to be placed against the adhesive, then pulled away slightly so that the adhesive can "set up" for a few minutes. One more caution: remember to wear protective eyewear when using a hammer, saw, or power tool.

Weight Room Construction

If you have space for a weight room, but don't have a separate room for equipment, you can easily build a wall or two that offers privacy. By simply building partitions (nonbearing walls), you can add your weight room, exercise room, gym, or other fitness room to your home or apartment.

Your partition framework should normally consist of 2 × 4 studs spaced 16 inches or 24 inches on center, nailed to a 2 × 4 sole plate at the floor line and corresponding 2 × 4 top plate at the ceiling. First lay out the wall's position on the floor with a chalk line, indicating openings for doors and location of any electrical boxes. Then cut 2 × 4s to length for sole and top plates and lay them side-by-side on the floor. Next, mark off stud locations on both pieces simultaneously to assure accuracy (Fig. 4-28).

Begin construction by nailing the sole plate to the floor if possible. Where the sole plate meets the wall, measure distance to the ceiling and subtract 1½ inches (the thickness of the top plate) to determine the length of the first stud. Cut this stud and toe-nail it to the sole plate. Use a level to make sure the stud is perfectly plumb, then nail it to the adjoining wall when permissible. Now slip the top plate into position above the stud and nail into the ceiling joist above. Finally, toe-nail the stud to the top plate. For toe-nailing, use 8d (2½-inch) nails at 60-degree angles, two to each side of the stud (except the one that's against the wall).

Continue to measure, plumb, and nail studs at 16-inch or 24-inch intervals. Use double studs at the sides and tops of any wall openings. When all framing is done, install required electrical wiring and attach electrical boxes to studs, as needed, setting them "out" sufficiently to allow for thickness of gypsum board and paneling. Finally, apply gypsum board sheets directly to the studs and cover

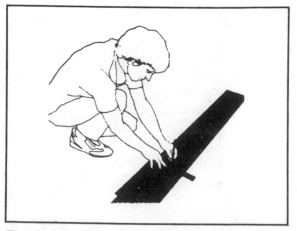

Fig. 4-28. Marking stud location. (Courtesy Georgia-Pacific)

with wall paneling and moldings of your choice.

If the preceding steps sound a bit complicated, there is an acceptable alternative that's simpler to do: build the partition flat on the floor then raise it into position so you can avoid toe-nailing. You nail directly up through the sole plate and down through the top plate into the ends of the studs. To provide clearance for raising the wall into position, you'll need to deduct 1 inch from the overall height. When in place, wedge the prebuilt wall firmly with wooden wedges under the sole plate, then nail securely into the ceiling joists, floor, and adjoining walls. Baseboard molding will cover the slight gap at the floor.

Temporary Fitness Center Walls

If you are an apartment dweller, a temporary wall may be the solution that allows you to redivide your living room, bedroom, or other space for a fitness room without nailing into the landlord's walls. In your own home, this can also provide for a future change as your fitness room grows.

Proceed with the prebuilt wall described earlier, but use 2 × 2 rather than 2 × 4 lumber. About every 4 feet in the top plate, drill ⅜-inch holes and insert t-nuts (small fasteners with internal screw threads) into the holes. Then insert ¼-inch carriage bolts, 2 inches long, into the t-nuts. Raise the wall into position and tighten the bolts using a small wrench. This will force the heads up against the ceiling (protect it with small paneling scraps) and push the wall firmly down against the floor. Done! Apply moldings at your discretion. If the wall is to be disassembled and moved in the future, build it in 4-foot sections and treat them as separate modules. Refer to Fig. 4-29.

Calculating Paneling Needs

Now that you've seen the different methods of

paneling a weight room or other fitness room wall, let's see how best to calculate your paneling needs to minimize waste. Begin by measuring the room and transferring those measurements to graph paper (Fig. 4-30). A graph diagram helps you visualize the project including the layout of the fitness equipment. If your room is 14 feet by 16 feet and each ¼-inch square on the graph paper equals 6 feet, you'll end up with a 7-inch-by-8-inch rectangle. Indicate windows, doors, and other structural elements. Now, total all wall widths and divide by 4 feet—the width of one panel. Refer to Table 4-1. If your total wall width falls between two numbers, "round up" to the highest

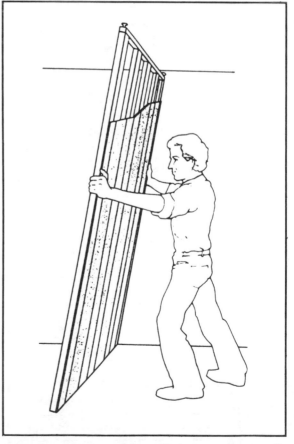

Fig. 4-29. Installing temporary walls for your temporary fitness room. (Courtesy Georgia-Pacific)

95

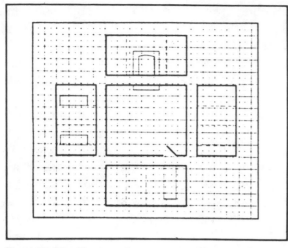

Fig. 4-30. Planning paneling on paper. (Courtesy Georgia-Pacific)

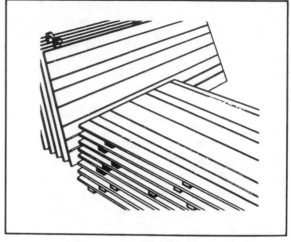

Fig. 4-31. Storing paneling. (Courtesy Georgia-Pacific)

number. As an example: 60 feet of wall requires sixteen 4-by-8-foot panels. However, 50 feet of wall needs 13 panels.

Store paneling in a dry location until it's ready to use. If walls are freshly plastered, allow them to dry thoroughly before installing paneling. Ideally, paneling should be stacked flat on the floor with spaced sticks between sheets to allow air circulation or propped on the 8-foot edge with sticks separating the sheets (Fig. 4-31). The panels should remain in the room 48 hours prior to installation to permit conditioning to the surrounding temperatures and humidity conditions.

The beauty of real wood paneling lies in the natural variety of grain and color displayed by each individual panel. Before you begin to install your paneling, take a few minutes to stand the panels side-by-side around the walls of the room. Now rearrange them to achieve

Table 4-1. Estimating Paneling.

Perimeter	No. of 4'x8' panels needed
36'	9
40'	10
44'	11
48'	12
52'	13
56'	14
60'	15
64'	16
68'	17
72'	18
92'	23

Courtesy Georgia-Pacific

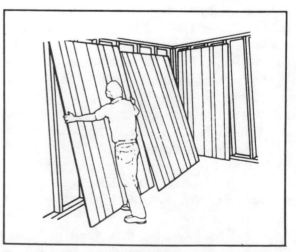

Fig. 4-32. Laying out paneling. (Courtesy Georgia-Pacific)

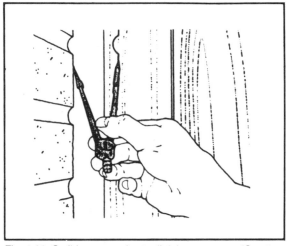

Fig. 4-33. Scribing a panel cut adjoining masonry. (Courtesy Georgia-Pacific)

the most pleasing balance of color and grain pattern, then number the back of each panel in sequence (Fig. 4-32). Be sure to note the grooving pattern as you arrange the panels to make sure you have the sequence of patterns you desire. Solutions to special paneling problems are offered in Figs. 4-33 through 4-36.

Your weight room is built and equipped. Let's take a look at building your own gym equipment in the next chapter.

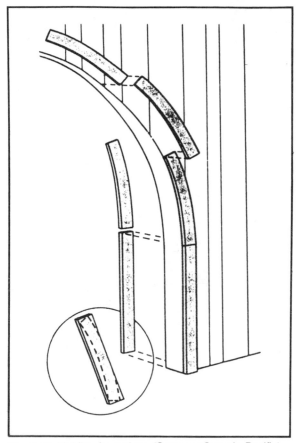

Fig. 4-35. Molding for arches. (Courtesy Georgia-Pacific)

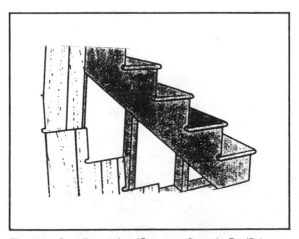

Fig. 4-34. Paneling stairs. (Courtesy Georgia-Pacific)

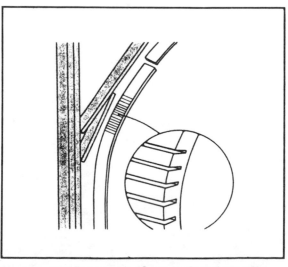

Fig. 4-36. Paneling an arch. (Courtesy Georgia-Pacific)

5

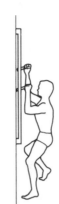

Gym Equipment

A GYM—SHORT FOR GYMNASIUM— IS A ROOM used for physical fitness. A gym can be anything from a place where boxers work out to a room specifically for gymnastics. In this chapter we'll look at gymnastics and how to build your own gymnastics equipment for fun and fitness.

Modern gymnastics exercises can be divided into two main groups: light gymnastics or calisthenics and heavy gymnastics. *Light gymnastics* is where most people begin and is intended primarily to develop muscle strength. Light gymnastics include knee bends, push-ups, kicks, headstands, and related activities. In a broad definition, light gymnastics can include exercises that gradually increase stress on muscles by using various devices such as dumbbells, and pulley weight machines as covered in the last chapter.

When most people think of gymnastics, however, they picture what is called heavy gymnastics. *Heavy gymnastics* emphasizes muscular control and coordination using fixed gymnasium equipment such as vaulting horses and mats, side horse, parallel bars, flying rings, horizontal bar, climbing ropes, horizontal and vertical ladders, and the trapeze. Mat gymnastics, such as cartwheels, handsprings, and related floor exercises, are also considered heavy gymnastics.

In the coming pages we'll offer instructions on how to plan and build some simple, yet useful heavy gymnastics equipment that can be used by gymnasts of all skill levels.

THE CLIMBER

The climber, also known as the wall climber or pegboard climber, is illustrated in Figs. 5-1 through 5-4. It is a very simple piece of equipment to build and use. It is mounted sturdily on a wall and the pegs are inserted into succes-

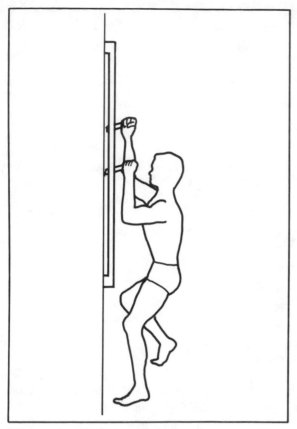

Fig. 5-1. Using the peg climber.

sively higher holes as you climb the wall. Using the climber will help build overall endurance and condition hand, arm, shoulder, and lower back muscles. Remember, if you decide to mount it outside, use waterproof adhesives and treat it against the elements.

Materials you need to construct the climber include a hardwood board 2 × 12 × 60 inches or as desired, two backing blocks ¾ × 2 × 12 inches of hardwood, and two climbing pegs 1⅛ inches in diameter by 9 inches long. The peg holes should be at an approximate 15-degree angle.

PARALLEL BARS

One of the most basic pieces of gymnastics equipment is the parallel bars. Figures 5-5 through 5-8 show the construction of low parallel bars, but you can easily adapt the design to fit your own needs.

Parallel bars are best built from welded one-inch steel pipe, but can be made of selected hardwood with simple modifications.

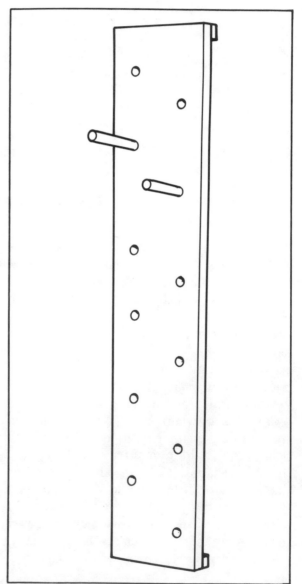

Fig. 5-2. Closeup of peg climber.

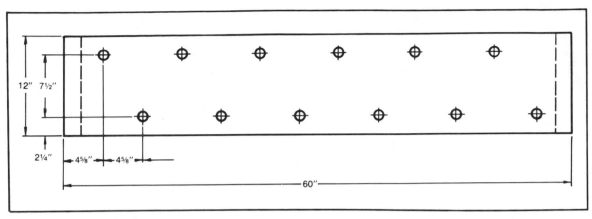

Fig. 5-3. Peg climber details.

You will need two rails, four legs, two feet, and four rubber or plastic protective tips.

A smaller version, called *pairoletts*, is illustrated in Figs. 5-9 through 5-12. They are used for developing hand balancing skills and are also built from welded steel. Materials needed include two rails, four legs, four feet, and eight feet tips.

VAULTING HORSE

The vaulting horse is another popular piece of gymnastics equipment that can be easily built. In official competition there are three types of vaulting horses: the men's horse (Fig. 5-13), the women's horse (smaller) and the pommel horse (Fig. 5-14).

The components are simple: the body, four legs, feet or cross-framing, and the pommels. For sturdy construction, use machine bolts and washers rather than nails. Make sure that there are no seams, nails, bolts, or other objects in any location where they could injure the vaulter.

ROPE CLIMB

A rope climb is an excellent exercise that offers versatility over the climber illustrated earlier. Yet a rope climb can be easily installed. Figure 5-15 illustrates the basic con-struction of a rope climb. The dimensions depend upon the height available. An outdoor rope climb is typically 10 to 15 feet tall, while an indoor climb will be limited to less than 8 feet in most cases. The disadvantage of the indoor rope climb can be overcome by beginning the climb in the sitting position rather than standing. Knots can be tied in the rope approximately every foot to offer a handhold and foothold. If you're using light rope, make sure you double or even triple it so it will be strong enough to hold two or more people for safety.

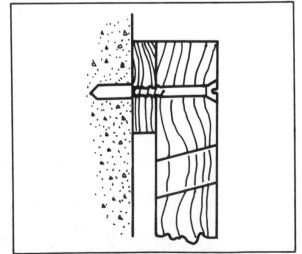

Fig. 5-4. Mounting the peg climber on a masonry wall.

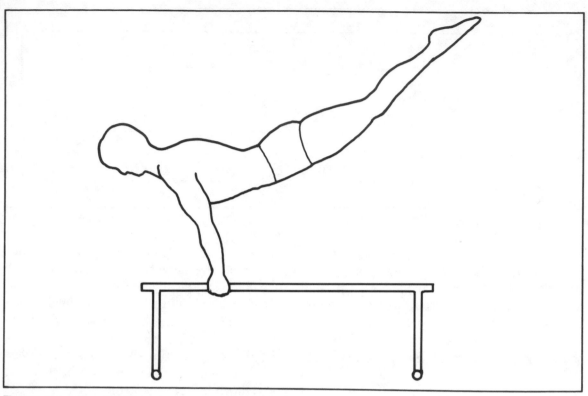

Fig. 5-5. Using the parallel bars.

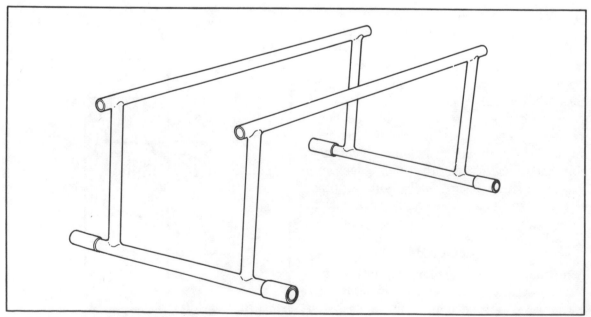

Fig. 5-6. Closeup of parallel bars.

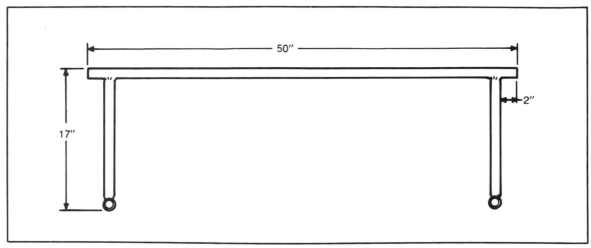

Fig. 5-7. Parallel bar detail.

RINGS

Figure 5-16 illustrates the construction of a ring. Two rings can be mounted in a gym room or on a special outdoor ring rig (Fig. 5-17). Rings can also be suspended from a tree limb or other object. Just make sure that it will support at least double your weight.

The ring itself can be made from steel or wood. Making one out of grained wood yourself, however, may be both difficult and unsafe.

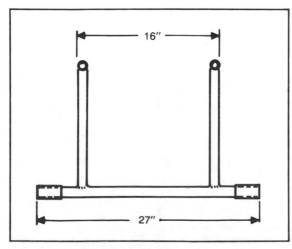

Fig. 5-8. End view of parallel bars.

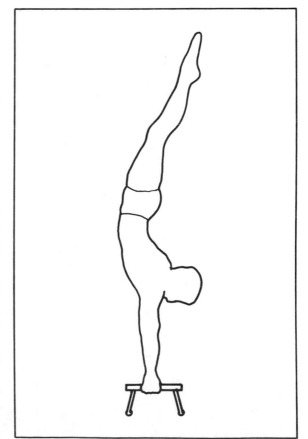

Fig. 5-9. Using the pairoletts.

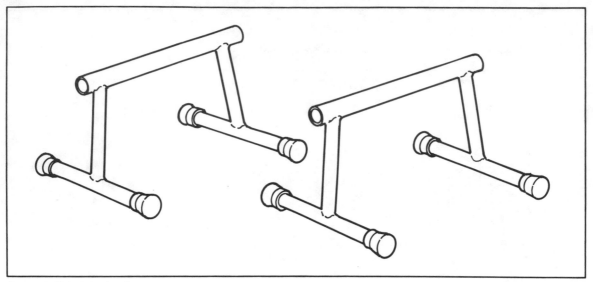

Fig. 5-10. Pairoletts detail.

A wooden ring would have to be made from 1-inch plywood. The framing can be of wood or steel as materials, budget, and skills dictate.

TRAPEZE

You can easily make a trapeze with a 1¼-inch steel rod or wood dowel hung by a chain (Fig. 5-18) or sturdy rope (Fig. 5-19). Again, the wood should be a hardwood and can be specially purchased or be made from an old, but sturdy, shovel handle. Drill two holes for the eye bolts, attach the chain top and bottom, and you can soon enjoy your trapeze.

Remember, though, that a trapeze requires more consideration for safety than many other pieces of gym equipment. Your entire

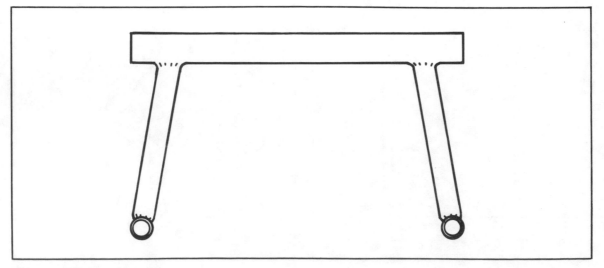

Fig. 5-11. Side view of pairoletts.

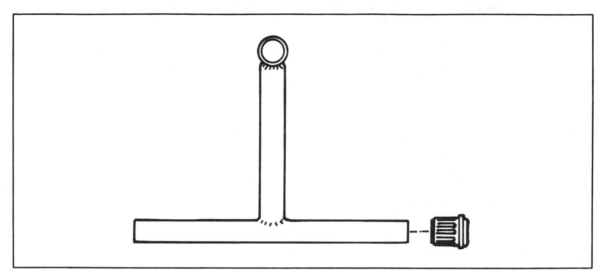

Fig. 5-12. End view of pairoletts.

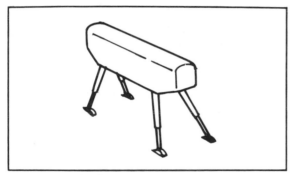

Fig. 5-13. Vaulting horse.

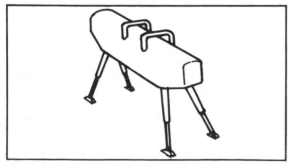

Fig. 5-14. Pommel horse.

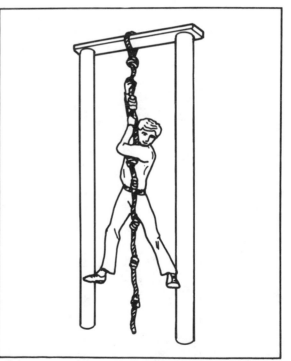

Fig. 5-15. Rope climb.

body weight will hang from the bar and attached supports, so you must be extra careful in selecting materials and in your installation.

HORIZONTAL LADDER

Both children and adults enjoy the horizontal ladder or "monkey bars" (Fig. 5-20). They are

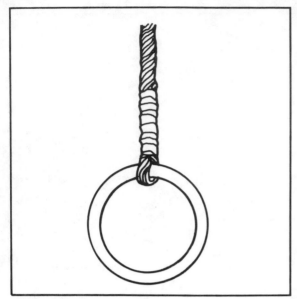

Fig. 5-16. Making your own ring.

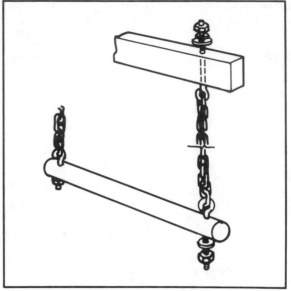

Fig. 5-18. Making a trapeze with pipe and chain.

easily constructed indoors or out and can help you build up shoulder and arm muscles enjoyably. The horizontal ladder can be incorporated into numerous other pieces of gym equipment, including the top climb, rings, trapeze, and the horizontal bar.

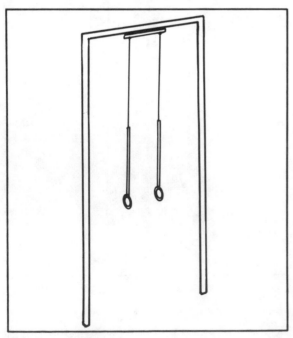

Fig. 5-17. Installing rings.

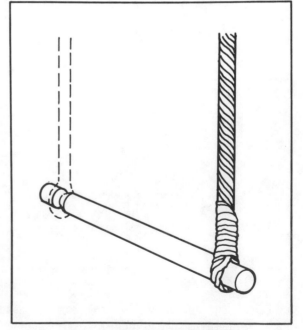

Fig. 5-19. Making a trapeze with wood and rope.

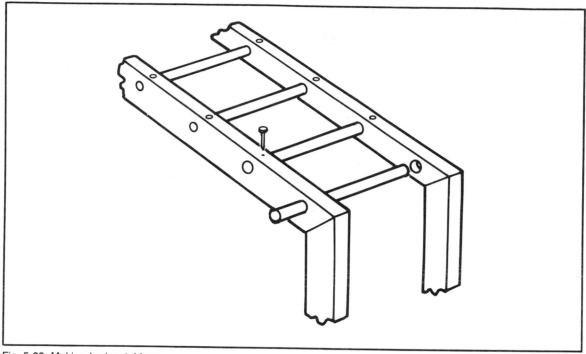

Fig. 5-20. Making horizontal bars.

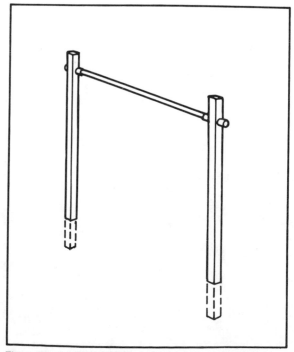

Fig. 5-21. Installing a horizontal bar rig into the ground.

The horizontal ladder can be built from 2 × 4s or 2 × 6s of good quality with 1¼-inch wooden dowels about 30 inches long. They are normally spaced about 1 foot apart, but can be as much as 18 inches apart for adults.

HORIZONTAL BAR

Figure 5-21 offers construction details for a typical horizontal bar that can be used for many exercises. Safety is important, so the horizontal bar must be supported by 4 × 4 posts anchored into the ground with cement or by using guy wires (Fig. 5-22). The bar itself is typically made of a 1½-inch to 2-inch pipe threaded and capped at both ends. As an additional safety feature, the pipe should be secured by a setscrew or dowel so that it doesn't roll in the gymnast's hands while being used.

Figure 5-23 shows the construction of asymmetrical bars that are popular with many women gymnasts. The bars can be base-

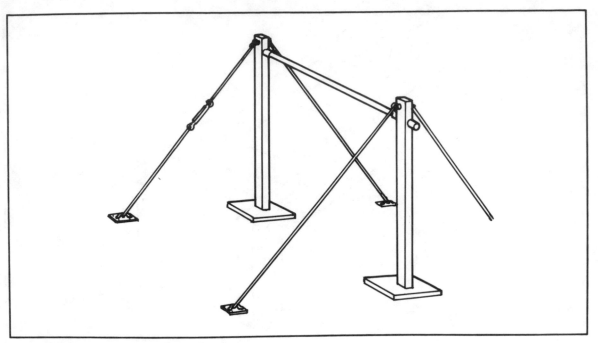

Fig. 5-22. Supporting horizontal bar with guy wires.

mounted or installed in concrete 2 or 3 feet below ground level. The frame can be of 4 × 4 posts and 1¼-inch water pipe or entirely of pipe and fittings. The turnbuckles add to the structural strength while allowing adjustment as needed.

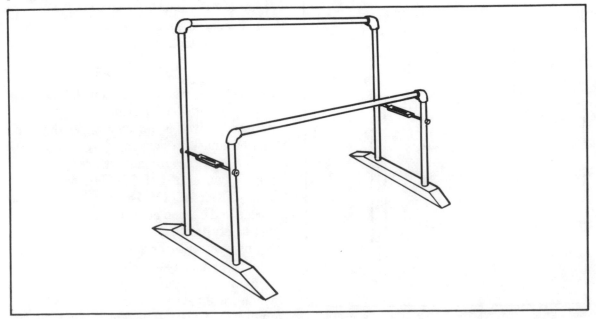

Fig. 5-23. Asymmetrical bars.

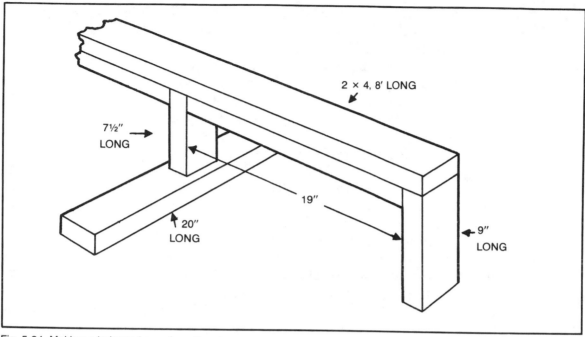

Fig. 5-24. Making a balance beam from 2 × 4s.

BALANCE BEAM

The balance beam is a simple, yet useful piece of gym equipment popular with both young and adult gymnasts. It can easily be constructed of wood and moved indoors or out as needed. Figure 5-24 shows the construction of a typical balance beam that can be built in a couple of hours.

There are many variations to the gym equipment shown in this chapter. Using these as guides, and following the construction techniques outlined in Chapter 2, you can easily adapt gym equipment to fit your personal needs and limitations.

SOUND INSULATION

Installing a gym or other fitness room in your home offers a variety of advantages to traveling to a public or private gym. It can also cause some problems, however, especially for those who don't share your enthusiasm for exercise or your timetable. Listening to the cadence grunts of an early bird exerciser can be distracting to sleepers and their consciences.

Room soundproofing can be the solution. In the next few pages we'll cover the basics of sound insulation and how you can apply them to your fitness room with a minimum of effort and expense. The ideas can be applied to new as well as existing construction.

HOW SOUND TRAVELS

How does sound travel and how is it transferred through a wall or floor? Airborne noises inside a room create sound waves which radiate outward from the source through the air until they strike a wall, floor, or ceiling. These surfaces are set in vibration by the fluctuating pressure of the sound wave in the air. Because the wall vibrates, it conducts sound to the other side in varying degrees, depending on the wall construction.

The resistance of a building element, such

as a wall, to the passage of airborne sound is rated by its *Sound Transmission Class* (STC). Thus the higher the number, the better the sound barrier. As an example, normal speech can be understood quite easily through a barrier with an STC 25 rating. If you must strain to hear the loud speech through a barrier, it is rated as an STC 45; and if loud speech is not audible through the barrier, it is an STC 50.

Sound travels readily through the air and also through some materials. When airborne sound strikes a conventional wall, the studs act as sound conductors unless they are separated in some way from the covering material. Electrical switches or convenience outlets placed back-to-back in a wall readily pass sound. Faulty construction, such as poorly fitted doors, often allows sound to travel through. Thus, good construction practices are important in providing sound-resistant walls, as well as those measures commonly used to stop ordinary sounds.

Thick walls of dense materials, such as masonry, can stop sound. But in the wood-frame house, an interior masonry wall results in increased costs and structural problems created by heavy walls. To provide a satisfactory sound-resistant wall economically has been a problem. At one time, sound-resistant frame construction for the home involved significant additional costs because it usually meant double walls or suspended ceilings. However, a relatively simple system has been developed using sound-deadening insulating board in conjunction with a gypsum board outer covering. This provides good sound-transmission resistance suitable for use in the home with only a slight additional cost. A number of combinations are possible with this system, providing different STC ratings.

WALL CONSTRUCTION

As noted earlier, a wall providing sufficient resistance to airborne sound transfer likely has an STC rating of 45 or greater. Thus in construction of such a wall between the rooms of a house, its cost as related to the STC rating should be considered. As shown in Fig. 5-25, detail *A* with gypsum wallboard and detail *B* with plastered wall are those commonly used for partition walls. The hypothetical rating of 45 cannot be obtained using this construction, however. An 8-inch concrete block wall (detail *C*) has the maximum rating, but this construction is not always practical in a wood-frame house.

Good STC ratings can be obtained in a wood-frame wall by using the combination of materials shown in *D* and *E*. One-half-inch sound-deadening board nailed to the studs, followed by a lamination of ½-inch gypsum wallboard, will provide an STC value of 46 at a relatively low cost. A slightly better rating can be obtained using ⅝-inch gypsum wallboard rather than ½-inch. A very satisfactory STC rating of 52 can be obtained by using resilient clips to fasten gypsum backer boards to the studs, followed by adhesive-laminated ½-inch fiberboard (*E*). This method further isolates the wall covering from the framing.

A similar isolation system consists of resilient channels nailed horizontally to 2 × 4 studs spaced 16 inches on center. Channels are spaced 24 inches apart vertically, and ⅝-inch gypsum wallboard is screwed to the channels. An STC rating of 47 is thus obtained at a moderately low cost.

The use of a double wall, which may consist of a 2 × 6 or wider plate and staggered 2-×-4-inch studs, is sometimes desirable. One-half-inch gypsum wallboard on each side of this wall (Fig. 5-26), detail *A*) results in an STC value of 45. However, two layers of ⅝-inch gypsum wallboard add little, if any, additional sound-transfer resistance (detail *B*). When 1½-inch blanket insulation is added to

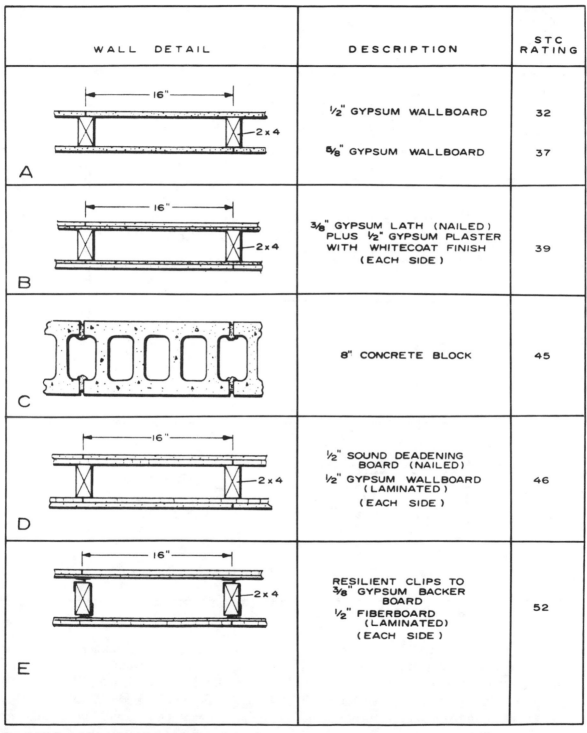

WALL DETAIL	DESCRIPTION	STC RATING
A	1/2" GYPSUM WALLBOARD	32
	5/8" GYPSUM WALLBOARD	37
B	3/8" GYPSUM LATH (NAILED) PLUS 1/2" GYPSUM PLASTER WITH WHITECOAT FINISH (EACH SIDE)	39
C	8" CONCRETE BLOCK	45
D	1/2" SOUND DEADENING BOARD (NAILED) 1/2" GYPSUM WALLBOARD (LAMINATED) (EACH SIDE)	46
E	RESILIENT CLIPS TO 3/8" GYPSUM BACKER BOARD 1/2" FIBERBOARD (LAMINATED) (EACH SIDE)	52

Fig. 5-25. Sound insulation of single walls.

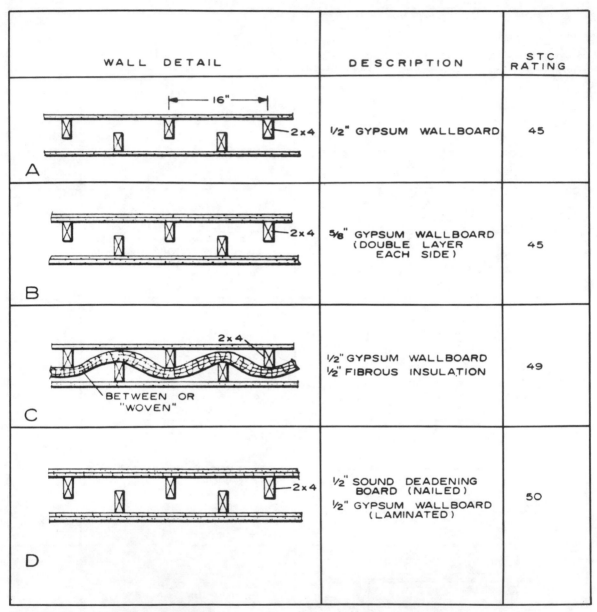

WALL DETAIL	DESCRIPTION	STC RATING
A 16" 2x4	1/2" GYPSUM WALLBOARD	45
B 2x4	5/8" GYPSUM WALLBOARD (DOUBLE LAYER EACH SIDE)	45
C 2x4 BETWEEN OR "WOVEN"	1/2" GYPSUM WALLBOARD 1/2" FIBROUS INSULATION	49
D 2x4	1/2" SOUND DEADENING BOARD (NAILED) 1/2" GYPSUM WALLBOARD (LAMINATED)	50

Fig. 5-26. Sound insulation of double walls.

this construction (*C*), the STC rating increases to 49. This insulation may be installed as shown or placed between studs on one wall. A single wall with 3½ inches of insulation will show a marked improvement over an open stud space and is low in cost.

The use of ½-inch sound-deadening board and a lamination of gypsum wallboard in the double wall will result in an STC rating of 50 (*D*). The addition of blanket insulation to this combination will likely provide an even higher value, perhaps 53 or 54.

FLOOR-CEILING SOUNDPROOFING

Sound insulation between an upper floor and the ceiling of a lower floor not only involves resistance of airborne sounds, but also that of impact noises. Impact noise control must therefore be considered as well as the STC value. *Impact noise* is caused by an object striking or sliding along a wall or floor surface, such as dropping objects, footsteps, or moving furniture. It may also be caused by the use of exercise or gymnastics equipment. In all instances, the floor is set into vibration by the

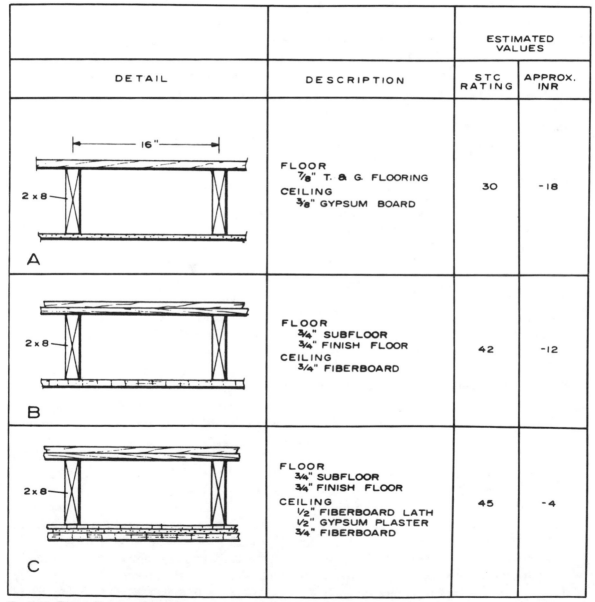

DETAIL	DESCRIPTION	ESTIMATED VALUES	
		STC RATING	APPROX. INR
A — 16" — 2 x 8	FLOOR ⅞" T. & G. FLOORING CEILING ⅜" GYPSUM BOARD	30	-18
B — 2 x 8	FLOOR ¾" SUBFLOOR ¾" FINISH FLOOR CEILING ¾" FIBERBOARD	42	-12
C — 2 x 8	FLOOR ¾" SUBFLOOR ¾" FINISH FLOOR CEILING ½" FIBERBOARD LATH ½" GYPSUM PLASTER ¾" FIBERBOARD	45	-4

Fig. 5-27. Floor-ceiling sound transfer.

impact or contact, and sound is radiated from both sides of the floor.

A method of measuring impact noise has been developed and is commonly expressed as the *Impact Noise Ratings* (INR). The greater the positive value of the INR, the more resistant is the floor to impact noise transfer. For example, an INR of −2 is better than one of −17, and one of +5 INR is a further improvement in resistance to impact noise transfer.

Figure 5-27 shows STC and approximate INR(db) values for several types of floor construction. Detail *A*, perhaps a minimum floor assembly with tongue-and-grooved floor and ⅜-inch gypsum board ceiling, has an STC value of 30 and an approximate INR value of −18. This is improved somewhat by the construction shown in detail *B*, and still further by the combination of materials in *C*.

The value of isolating the ceiling joists from a gypsum lath and plaster ceiling by means of spring clips is illustrated in Fig. 5-28, detail *A*. An STC value of 52 and an approximate INR value of −2 results.

Foam rubber padding and carpeting improve both the STC and the INR values. The STC value increases from 31 to 45 and the approximate INR from −17 to +5 (details *B* and *C*). This can likely be further improved by using an isolated ceiling finish with spring clips. The use of sound-deadening board and a lamination of gypsum board for the ceiling would also improve resistance to sound transfer.

An economical construction similar to (but better than) detail *C*, with an STC value of 48 and an approximate INR of +18, consists of the following:

- ☐ A pad and carpet over ⅝-inch tongue-and-grooved plywood underlayment,
- ☐ 3-inch fiberglass insulating batts between joists.

- ☐ resilient channels spaced 24 inches apart, across the bottom of the joists, and
- ☐ ⅝-inch gypsum board screwed to the bottom of the channels and finished with taped joints.

The use of separate floor joists with staggered ceiling joists below provides reasonable values but adds a good deal of construction costs. Separate joists with insulation between and a soundboard between floor and finish provide an STC rating of 53 and an approximate INR value of −3.

SOUND ABSORPTION

Design of the "quiet" room or house can incorporate another system of sound insulation, namely, sound absorption. Sound-absorbing materials can minimize the amount of noise by stopping the reflection of sound back into a room. Sound-absorbing materials do not necessarily have resistance to airborne sounds.

Perhaps the most commonly used sound-absorbing material is acoustic tile. Wood fiber or similar materials are used in the manufacture of the tile, which is usually processed to provide some fire resistance and designed with numerous tiny sound traps on the tile surfaces. This can consist of tiny drilled or punched holes, fissured surfaces, or a combination of both.

Acoustic tile is most often used in the ceiling and areas where it is not subjected to excessive mechanical damage, such as above a wall wainscoting. It is normally manufactured in sizes from 12 by 12 to 12 by 48 inches. Thicknesses vary from ½ to ¾ inch, and the tile is usually factory-finished ready for application. Paint or other finishes that fill or cover the tiny holes or fissures for trapping sound will greatly reduce its efficiency.

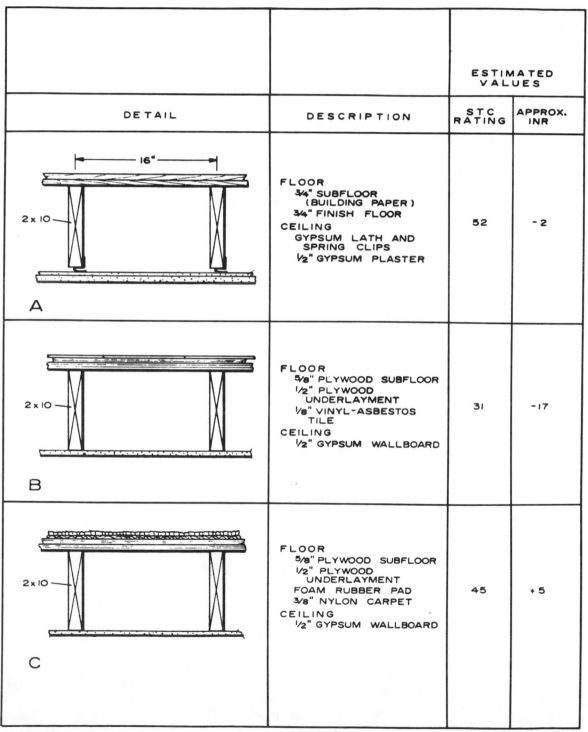

DETAIL	DESCRIPTION	ESTIMATED VALUES	
		STC RATING	APPROX. INR
A	FLOOR ¾" SUBFLOOR (BUILDING PAPER) ¾" FINISH FLOOR CEILING GYPSUM LATH AND SPRING CLIPS ½" GYPSUM PLASTER	52	- 2
B	FLOOR ⅝" PLYWOOD SUBFLOOR ½" PLYWOOD UNDERLAYMENT ⅛" VINYL-ASBESTOS TILE CEILING ½" GYPSUM WALLBOARD	31	- 17
C	FLOOR ⅝" PLYWOOD SUBFLOOR ½" PLYWOOD UNDERLAYMENT FOAM RUBBER PAD ⅜" NYLON CARPET CEILING ½" GYPSUM WALLBOARD	45	+ 5

Fig. 5-28. Floor-ceiling sound transfer.

Acoustic tile can be applied, by a number of methods, to existing ceilings or any smooth surface using a mastic adhesive designed specifically for this purpose or to furring strips nailed to the underside of the ceiling joists. Nailing or stapling tile is the normal application method in this system. It is also used with a mechanical suspension system involving small "H," "Z," or "T" members. Your local paint and tile store can give you more information on which acoustic tile to select and how to apply it with simple skills and tools.

Barriers of 4-×-8-foot sheets of plywood can be covered with acoustic tile and used as portable sound barriers for those in apartments or who must share room with others while exercising.

Sound insulation can give you peace of mind that your fitness program is not frustrating others around you.

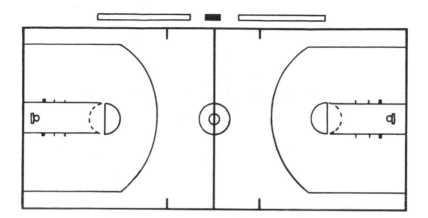

6

Build Your Own Indoor Courts

T HOSE WHO BECOME COURT SPORTS ENTHU-
siasts·—basketball, handball, racquetball,
tennis, badminton—soon begin dreaming of
having their own private courts where play
time is always available and no appointments
are necessary. For most, this dream remains
so.

But for some, private indoor courts are a
reality. The rich? Yes, but also some of the
not-so-rich who have a love for their sport
strong enough to take the time and money
needed to do it themselves. Simple, yet useful
courts can be set up in large unused rooms,
remodeled garages, or even special buildings.
It's all very possible and, for many, quite practical.

In this chapter you'll consider how to install a few of these courts yourself—complete
with markings—in existing or new space.
Continuing our do-it-all-yourself program,
you'll learn how to paint fitness rooms, courts,

and equipment. Many more outdoor courts will
be covered in Chapter 9.

PLANNING

Indoor sports courts require a great deal more
room than a simple exercise area or fitness
room. Most of us don't have this space readily
available, but have to develop it through planning and spending. Costs do not have to be
prohibitive. Let's consider a few ways of effectively planning your indoor court.

First, consider what space you have cur-
rently available for such a court. General dimensions will be given later. In most cases,
courts are often larger than typical room size.
Consider places like unused basements, garages, or outbuildings such as barns. Look
carefully. Many types of sports courts can be
marked out in a double garage allowing fitness
fun when the car(s) are driven out. Low basement ceilings are a problem with many types of

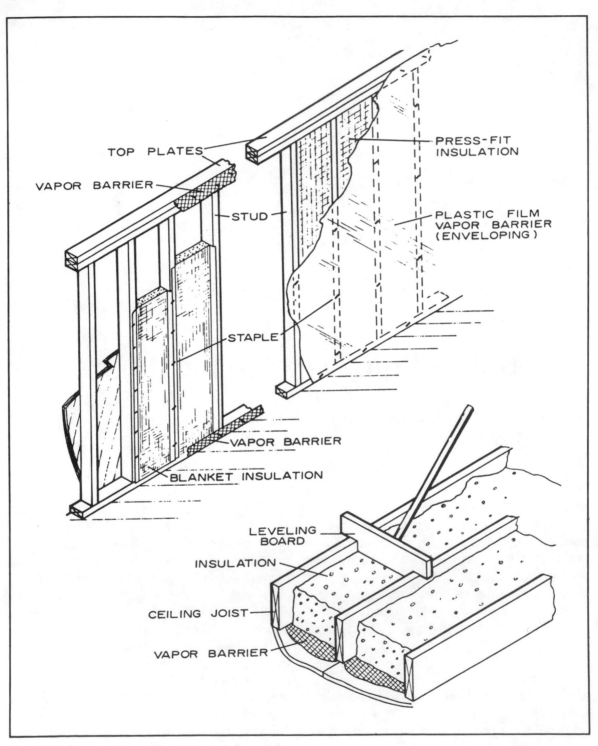

Fig. 6-1. Wall construction and insulation for indoor courts.

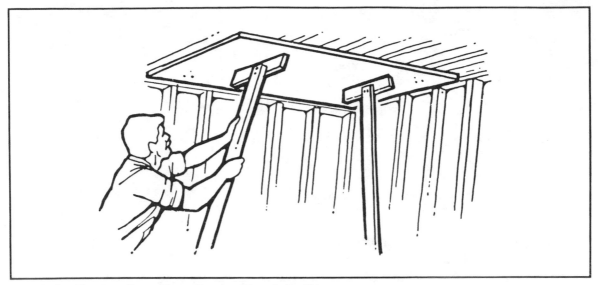

Fig. 6-2. Installing drywall on ceilings. (Courtesy Georgia-Pacific)

courts, but if you're planning a shuffleboard court, they can be easily modified in many cases. Barns and other outbuildings can house sports courts with slight modifications, depending on the building. If you're really into your game, a pole building can be used to enclose many types of indoor and outdoor courts (Figs. 6-1 through 6-10).

Don't give up yet, you may be able to find others in your neighborhood who share your enthusiasm for indoor sports and either have the available space or are willing to share the costs of setting a court up. Get it down on paper and give it a try.

HANDBALL COURTS

Handball and racquetball courts are becoming the most popular indoor sports courts. They offer year-round recreation for men, women, and children with minimal equipment required

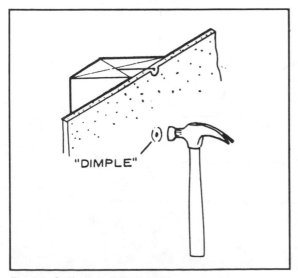

Fig. 6-3. Setting a nail in drywall.

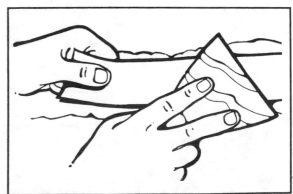

Fig. 6-4. Taping drywall. (Courtesy Georgia-Pacific)

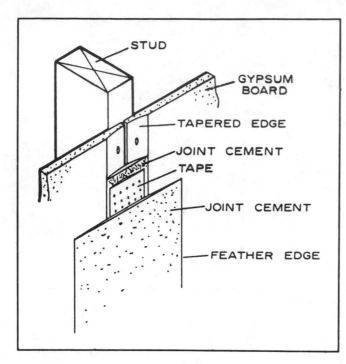

STUD

GYPSUM BOARD

TAPERED EDGE

JOINT CEMENT

TAPE

JOINT CEMENT

FEATHER EDGE

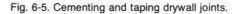
Fig. 6-5. Cementing and taping drywall joints.

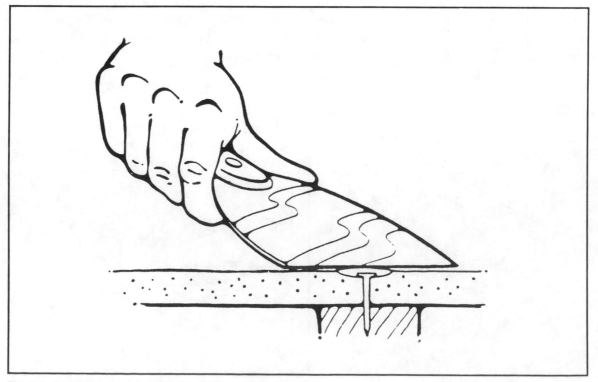

Fig. 6-6. Cementing drywall nailheads. (Courtesy Georgia-Pacific)

120

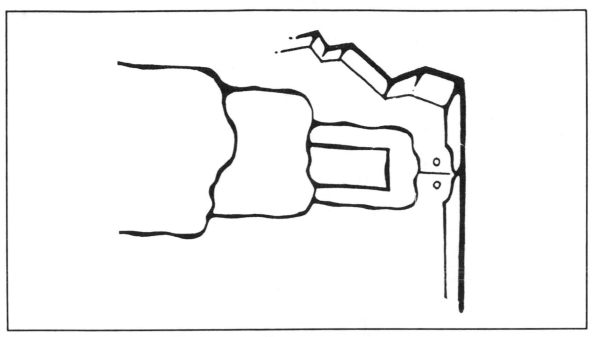

Fig. 6-7. Drywall taping and finishing coats. (Courtesy Georgia-Pacific)

once the court is established. Figure 6-11 illustrates the layout of a three-wall handball court and Fig. 6-12 shows the same for a four-wall court, as suggested by the United States Handball Association.

For a four-wall handball court you'll need about 800 square feet; a three-wall court requires about 1000 square feet. While these are large courts, you can certainly modify the dimensions to fit your own *un*official needs. Such

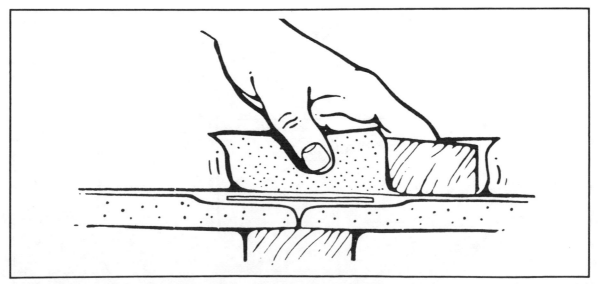

Fig. 6-8. Smoothing drywall seams with sandpaper. (Courtesy Georgia-Pacific)

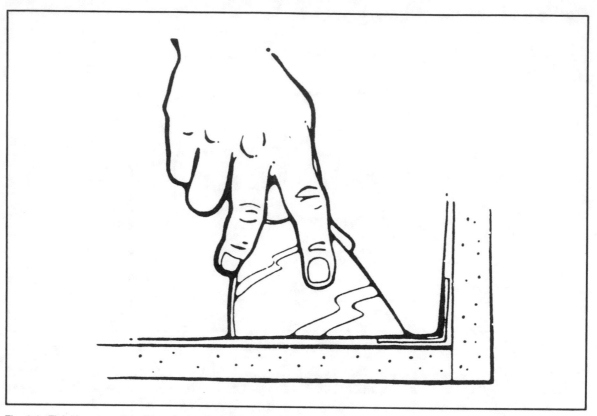

Fig. 6-9. Finishing drywall inside corner. (Courtesy Georgia-Pacific)

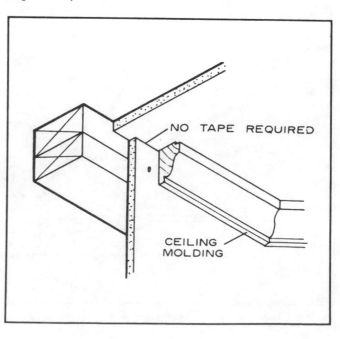

Fig. 6-10. Finishing drywall at ceiling.

NO TAPE REQUIRED

CEILING MOLDING

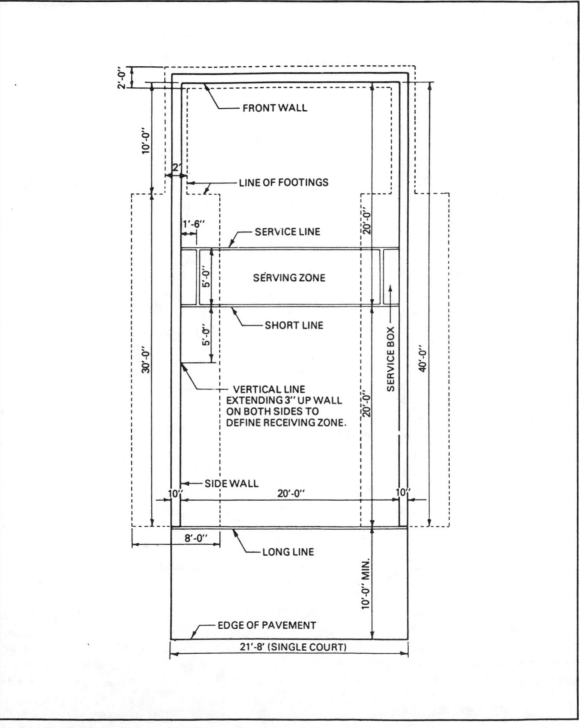

FRONT WALL

LINE OF FOOTINGS

SERVICE LINE

SERVING ZONE

SHORT LINE

VERTICAL LINE
EXTENDING 3'' UP WALL
ON BOTH SIDES TO
DEFINE RECEIVING ZONE.

SIDE WALL

LONG LINE

EDGE OF PAVEMENT

SERVICE BOX

2'-0''
10'-0''
2'
1'-6''
5'-0''
5'-0''
30'-0''
20'-0''
20'-0''
40'-0''
10''
20'-0''
10''
8'-0''
10'-0'' MIN.
21'-8' (SINGLE COURT)

Fig. 6-11. Three-wall handball court layout.

123

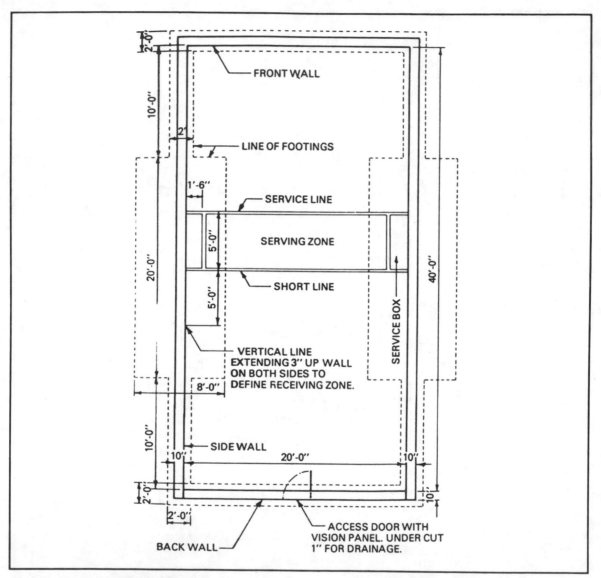

Fig. 6-12. Four-wall handball court layout.

a handball court can easily be set up in your garage or high-ceiling basement for hours of fun and fitness. These courts can also be taken outdoors if your backyard and the weather are agreeable.

BASKETBALL COURTS

One of America's favorite games is basketball. It's played in every city, community, school, and driveway. Many want to have their own indoor basketball court at home. The size of "official" courts prohibits most from erecting such a court, but a few set them up in outbuildings. Many play "half court" or otherwise modify the dimensions of the standard basketball court.

124

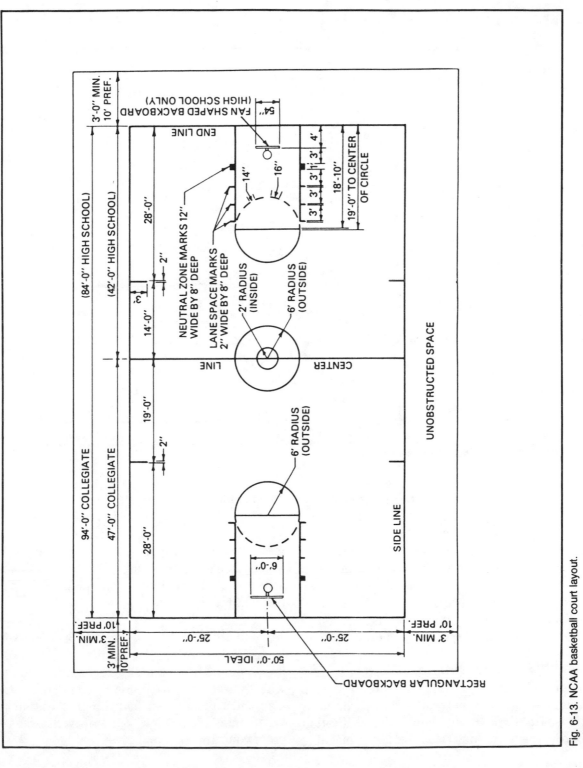

Fig. 6-13. NCAA basketball court layout.

125

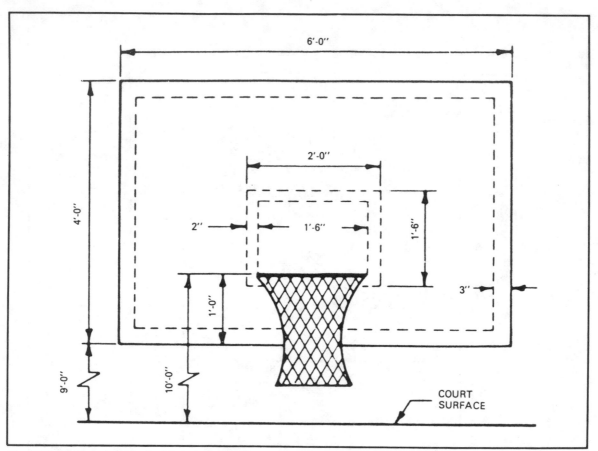

Fig. 6-14. NCAA rectangular backboard construction.

Figure 6-13 illustrates the dimensions of a court as established by the NCAA or National Collegiate Athletic Association. Included are dimensions for both high school and collegiate play. Figure 6-14 shows the construction of the standard rectangular backboard. Figure 6-15 shows the construction of a fan-shaped backboard as used in many high schools. These, too, can be easily installed outdoors.

TENNIS, BADMINTON, AND OTHER COURTS

There are numerous types of outdoor sports courts that can be moved indoors if you have the space. Rather than cover each modification here, take what you've learned about planning and installing indoor courts and apply it to the sports courts and facilities suggested in Chapter 9. Nearly all of them can be brought indoors with some planning, sizing, and hard work. Don't let your dreams of a personal sports court be limited by anything less than true limitations.

PAINTING ROOMS AND COURTS

In earlier chapters you've learned to select and use tools, develop building techniques, work with contractors, make your own equipment, plan and build rooms, and remodel garages, basements, and other rooms—even sound-proof your fitness room. Now you'll learn how to paint rooms, courts, and equipment so they will be both decorative and more practical.

The subject of painting is a large one, and different situations are constantly encountered by the do-it-yourselfer which are not covered in the basics. When this happens, the best thing to do is consult an experienced paint dealer or contractor before going ahead with the job. Never apply paint to a surface until you are certain of the results. The application of paint takes only a short time, but removing it is a difficult job.

Good results in painting depend upon the selection and care of brushes and other tools, the selection and mixing of the paint, and the proper preparation of the surface to be painted. Unless these three factors are fully considered, the hours and money spent will probably be wasted.

PAINT BRUSHES

The importance of buying only the best grade of paint brush cannot be overstressed. A poor quality brush will not only deteriorate quickly and have to be replaced, but will not produce good work while still in usable condition. A good brush must be properly cared for like any other good tool. It will last through many jobs and always give good results.

Figure 6-16 illustrates the components of

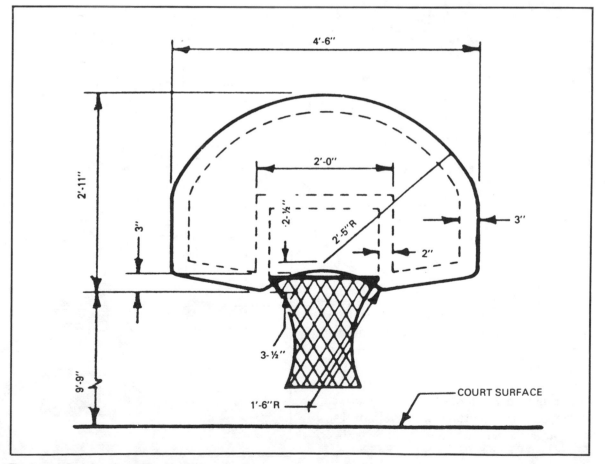

Fig. 6-15. NCAA fan-shaped backboard construction.

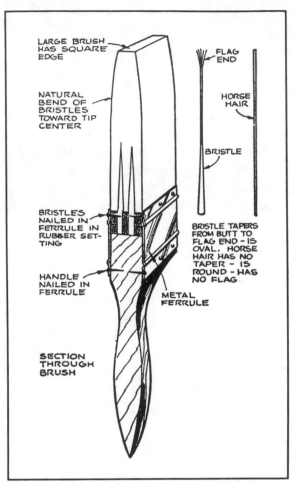

Fig. 6-16. Construction of a flat paint brush.

wall brush is the best. These come in several sizes, but a brush 4 inches wide with the bristles 4 or more inches long is excellent for most jobs. Small woodwork, such as interior trim and exterior work, requires a flat trim or sash brush. These vary from 1 to 3 inches in width and are similar in shape to the flat wall brush. An oval sash brush with a chisel end is excellent for working around windows and for other difficult places.

A paint brush should never be used for varnish, although a brush that has been used for varnish can be used for paint. Why? The reason is that it is almost impossible to remove every trace of paint from a brush. If a brush

a good paint brush—a flat brush. There is a paint brush for almost every kind of job, but it isn't necessary to have a full collection to get good results for your work. A good brush, neither too large nor too small, can be used for many jobs. A painter uses a wide brush on large surfaces rather than a small brush which would require many more strokes to cover the same area.

Figure 6-17 shows five of the more common types of paint brushes: flat wall, oval sash, angular sash and trim, duster, and woodwork. Figure 6-18 illustrates a calcimine brush. For house painting or for other large surfaces, a flat

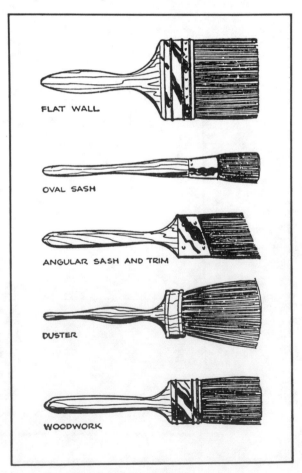

Fig. 6-17. Common paint brush types.

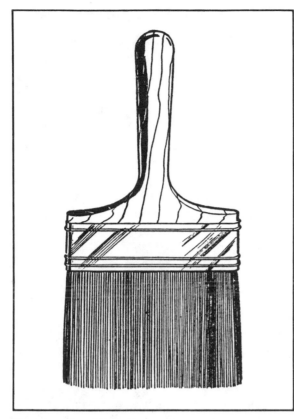

Fig. 6-18. Flat calcimine brush.

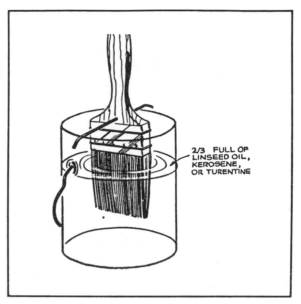

Fig. 6-19. Storing a brush.

containing a small amount of paint is dipped into varnish, the paint will discolor the clear varnish enough to spoil the effect. It is best to keep one brush for varnish only. There are special brushes for varnishing which have a tapered end, permitting the varnish to flow easily.

Once you've purchased a good brush, take proper care of it. Figure 6-19 depicts the best method of storing a paint brush for a short period, such as overnight. If you must store it longer, thoroughly clean and wrap it as shown in Fig. 6-20.

Spray Painting

Spray painting is also popular for large surfaces such as walls and doors. Care must be taken to minimize overspray, however. Figure 6-21 shows the common spray gun with attached paint container. Details of a more professional spray gun are shown in Fig. 6-22. Figure 6-23 gives the flow in an external mix spray head that offers a good spray pattern for the general painting jobs.

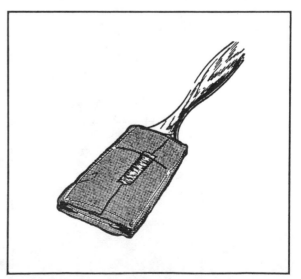

Fig. 6-20. Wrapping a paint brush for storage.

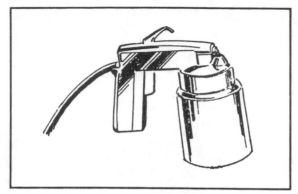

Fig. 6-21. Spray gun with attached cup.

Rollers and Pads

Paint rollers and painting pads are increasingly popular for do-it-yourself painting. They are easy to use, spread quickly, and clean up easily. One of the most important considerations is the quality of the tools and paint. Cheap painting tools and cheap paint show up more using rollers and pads than they do with paint brushes.

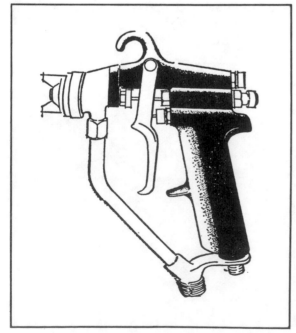

Fig. 6-22. Pressure spray gun.

Selecting Paints

There are two basic kinds of paint used around the home. One is called oil-based or solvent-thinned paint which is composed of a pigment such as white lead with linseed oil used as the vehicle. The other is water-based or water-thinned paint—commonly called "latex" paint—in which a whiting and glue are mixed with a water vehicle.

Exterior or house paints are made for all surfaces exposed to the weather and to extreme changes in temperature. It can be applied to wood or metal provided the metal has been properly treated before the paint is applied.

Interior oil paint is similar to that used for outside work except that it is not as resistant to moisture and temperature changes. It should, however, be sufficiently tough and durable to withstand washings and to keep moisture from penetrating to the woodwork.

Latex paint is the most popular for interior work. For better quality latex paint, at least 50 percent of the pigment binder should be latex solids. The main ingredient in the pigment should be titanium dioxide, the ingredient that provides covering up or hiding ability, with the ingredients specified by weight and not by volume.

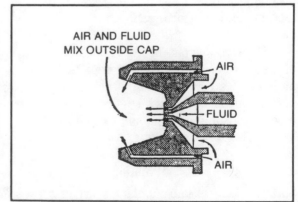

Fig. 6-23. External-mix spray head.

Using Paints

Latex paints can be applied over sheet rock or plaster walls once the walls are dry. But keep in mind that taped joints of Sheetrock® are basically a wet material and, like a plastered wall, should "cure" for about two weeks before the surface coating is applied.

Another precaution comes from the paint can label, and this gives the number of square feet one gallon will cover. If the label indicates that the gallon will cover 450 square feet, then do not exceed this. If you do, the result will be unsatisfactory. In fact, you might see weak spots in the paint film even though the guarantee states the paint will cover in one coat. For truly satisfactory results, apply two coats of latex paint. Always make sure that the paint is *thoroughly* mixed.

Surface Preparation

Paint can only be applied to a clean surface (Fig. 6-24). Grease and dirt should be completely removed by washing the surface with water and a nonsoapy cleaner, as soap leaves a thin film on the surface to interfere with the paint. A cloth soaked in turpentine can be used to wipe off a surface before painting. If the surface has been previously painted, and the paint is still in good condition, cleaning is all that is necessary before applying the new coat. If the old paint has cracked or blistered, scrape or sand it off.

Moisture will spoil any painted surface. The surface must be absolutely dry with no possibility of the moisture seeping through from the opposite side and penetrating beneath the paint. After a rain, no outside painting

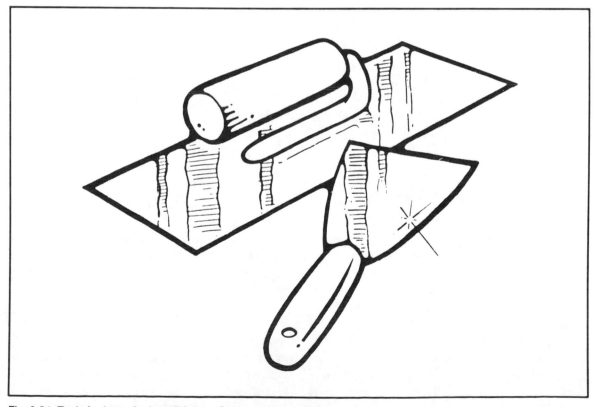

Fig. 6-24. Tools for brocade drywall finish. (Courtesy Georgia-Pacific)

should be done for several days so that the wood will dry completely. It is equally important not to do any outside painting in the early morning when there is dew on the surface or late in the afternoon or early evening when the dew is gathering. Temperature must be considered as well. Don't attempt to paint if the temperature is less than 50° F as the cold will cause the paint to thicken and not flow properly. It is a waste of time and money to paint when conditions are not favorable.

Old paint can be removed from wood by several methods. For small jobs, a hand scraper and sandpaper can be used. The blade should be sharp, and care should be taken not to let a corner of it gouge into the wood—or you.

A liquid paint remover is one that will soften the paint or varnish so that it may be scraped and wiped off the surface with moderate ease. To use, brush the liquid over the surface and allow it to remain until the paint begins to soften. After the paint has been removed, the surface should be wiped with alcohol to remove all traces of the remover. Don't use a liquid paint and varnish remover in an unventilated room or one in which there is an open flame.

To remove large quantities of old paint, many professional painters use a blowtorch together with a broad putty knife. The flame of the torch softens the paint which can then be easily removed with the scraper. There are a few simple precautions to be observed when using a blowtorch. It should be pointed down, never up. Don't allow the flame of the torch to become too hot or it may char the wood. When working on the outside of the house, make sure there are no birds' nests or other flammable matter under the eaves.

Some communities forbid the use of a blowtorch for removing paint, so consult local authorities before beginning work. Likewise,

consult with your insurance agent to find out whether there is any clause in your home fire insurance policy that forbids work of this nature.

Brush Painting

To paint with a brush, first select the type of brush and paint pot needed for the job as discussed. The best type of paint pot for brush painting is a 1-gallon paint can from which the lip around the top has been removed (Fig. 6-25). Dip the brush to only one-third the length of the bristles. Scrape the surplus paint off the lower face of the brush so there will be no drip as you transfer the brush from the pot to the work.

Figure 6-26 shows how to apply paint by brush on larger surfaces. *Laying on* means applying the paint first in long, horizontal strokes. *Laying off* means crossing your first strokes by working up and down. By using the laying on and laying off method and crossing your strokes, the paint is distributed evenly over the surface, the surface is completely covered, and a minimum amount of paint is used. A good rule is to "lay on" the paint the shortest distance across the area and "lay off" the longest distance. When painting walls or any vertical surface, "lay on" in horizontal strokes, "lay off" vertically.

Always paint ceilings first and work from the far corner. By working the ceiling first, you can keep the wall free of drippings by wiping up as you go. When painting ceiling surfaces, "lay on" paint coats for the shortest ceiling distance and "lay off" for the longest ceiling distance.

To avoid brush marks when finishing up a square, use strokes directed toward the last square finished, gradually lifting the brush near the end of the stroke while the brush is still in motion. Every time the brush touches the painted surface at the start of a stroke, it leaves a mark. For this reason, never finish a

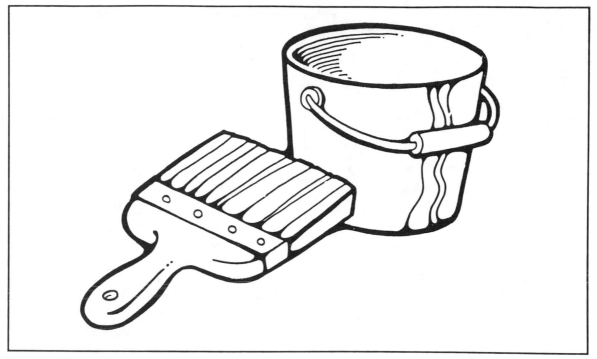

Fig. 6-25. Paint brush and bucket. (Courtesy Georgia-Pacific)

square by brushing toward the unpainted area, but always end up by brushing back toward the area already painted. Always carry a rag for wiping dripped or smeared paint.

Roller Painting

To paint with a roller and tray (Fig. 6-27), pour the premixed paint into the tray to about one-half the depth of the tray. Immerse the roller completely, then roll it back and forth along the ramp to fill the cover completely and remove any excess paint. As an alternative to using the tray, place a specially designed galvanized wire screen into a five-gallon can of paint. The screen attaches to the can and remains at the correct angle for loading and spreading paint on the roller.

The first load of paint on a roller should be worked out on newspaper to remove entrapped air from the roller cover. It is then ready for application. As the roller is passed over a surface, thousands of tiny fibers continually compress and expand, metering out the coating and wetting the surface.

Always trim around ceilings, moldings,

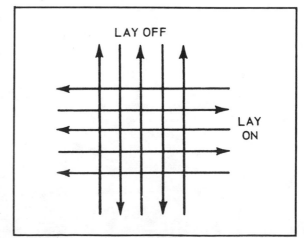

Fig. 6-26. Laying on and laying off.

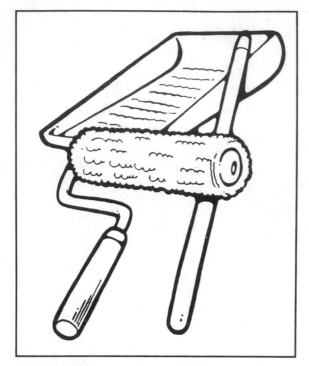

Fig. 6-27. Paint roller and pan. (Courtesy Georgia-Pacific)

paint onto the surface, working from the dry area into the just-painted area. Never roll completely in the same or one direction. Don't roll too fast and avoid spinning the roller at the end of the stroke. Always feather out final strokes to pick up any excess paint on the surface. This is done by rolling the final stroke out with minimal pressure.

Spray Painting Methods

Figure 6-28 shows the correct method of stroking with a spray gun. Hold the gun 6 to 8 inches from the surface to be painted, keep the axis of the spray perpendicular to the surface, and take strokes back and forth in horizontal lines. Pull the trigger just after you start a stroke to avoid applying too much paint at the starting and stopping points.

Figure 6-29 shows the right and wrong methods of spraying an outside corner. If you use the wrong method shown, a good deal of paint will be wasted into the air through overspray.

Painting Safety

A variety of ingredients used in manufacture of

etc., before rolling the major wall or ceiling surfaces. Then roll as close as possible to maintain the same texture. Trimming is usually done with a 3-inch wall brush. Always roll

Fig. 6-28. Correct method of stroking with a spray gun.

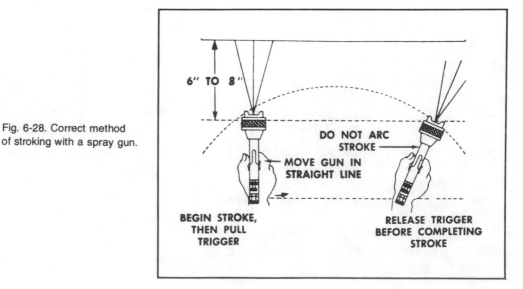

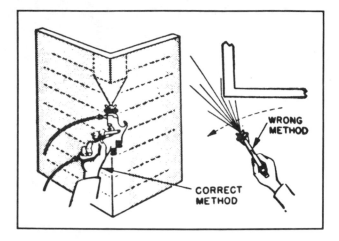

Fig. 6-29. Right and wrong methods of spraying outside corner.

paint materials are injurious to the human body in varying degrees. While the body can withstand nominal quantities of most of these poisons for relatively short periods of time, continuous or overexposure to them may have harmful effects. Nevertheless, health hazards can easily be avoided by a common sense approach of avoiding unnecessary contact with hazardous materials:

☐ Make sure toxic materials are properly identified and kept tightly sealed when not in use.
☐ Make sure equipment is in good condition and working properly, especially spray guns and ladders.

☐ Make sure that ventilation is adequate and use a respirator if necessary.
☐ Wear safety equipment such as goggles and a filter mask when painting or sandblasting.
☐ Wear gloves when handling toxic materials.
☐ Avoid touching any part of the body, especially the face, when handling paints and related materials. Wash hands and face thoroughly before eating and at the end of the day.

Think carefully about safety and efficiency as you paint your fitness room, court, or equipment.

135

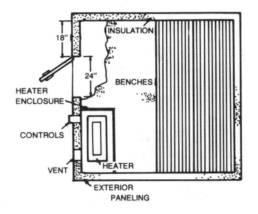

7

Sauna

T HE SAUNA HAS BEEN A FAVORITE OF PEO-
ple interested in fitness for many years. In
fact, the Finns say their sauna dates back over
two thousand years. The turkish bath is about
as old.

The purpose of the sauna is to cleanse the
body through perspiration. That is, dry heat is
used to encourage the body to sweat and pass
perspiration through the skin's pores and flush
out impurities.

The sauna is simply a wood-walled room
with a stove that heats rocks which, in turn,
heat up the room's air to make the bather
perspire. There are many variations to this
simple formula. Saunas can be built in conjunction with a hot tub, swimming pool, or other
body of water where a quick dunking can be
enjoyed immediately after by the hearty.

Today, saunas are built either indoors or
outdoors, permanent or portable, depending
on the needs and the budget of the builder.

Many sauna kits are available for building
free-standing saunas outdoors or converting a
bathroom or corner of the garage into a
sauna—with or without an adjoining shower or
changing room.

PLANNING

Figure 7-1 illustrates the layout of a typical
sauna. Figure 7-2 shows a side view of the
same sauna. As you can see, about half of the
floor space is taken up by benches where two
to six people can lay or sit to enjoy their sauna.
The heater is typically located in the corner of
the sauna room and controls are on the outside
of the door.

Saunas can be built to nearly any size.
Common sizes include 3 by 3 (solo), 4 by 6, 6
by 6, 6 by 9, and 6 by 12 feet. Most have
headroom of approximately 6 feet 8 inches.
Smaller saunas can be heated with 110-volt
heaters, while larger units require 220-volt

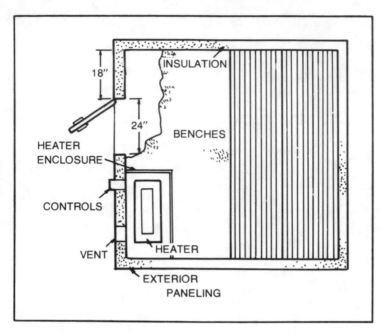

Fig. 7-1. Sauna plan view.

wiring to operate. Keep this in mind as you plan the size, location, and requirements of your sauna. Heaters are usually small: 14 inches square and 24 inches high to 24 inches square by 24 inches high.

BUILDING

A free-standing sauna can be built indoors or outdoors, depending on the space available and your interest in braving the elements year-round in order to enjoy it. An outdoor free-standing sauna can easily be built using construction techniques outlined in Chapter 2. The foundation can be simply of piers set on concrete poured into holes in the ground, or it can be more elaborate for larger units. Most are built on simple concrete blocks for economy and ease of movement.

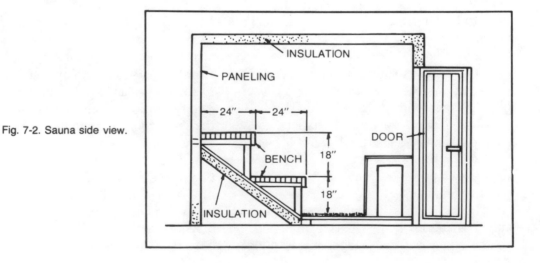

Fig. 7-2. Sauna side view.

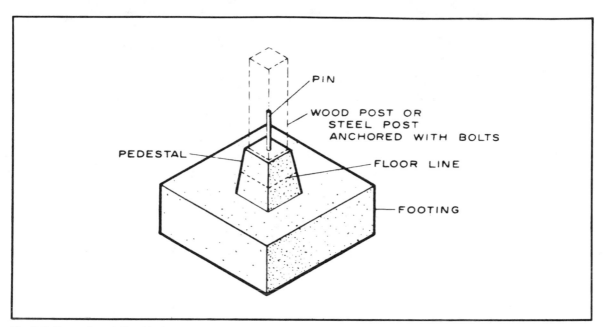

Fig. 7-3. Sauna foundation block.

Figure 7-3 shows a typical foundation for a small building such as an outdoor free-standing sauna. The subflooring is then installed and the walls are erected. Figures 7-4 through 7-9 and Table 7-1 illustrate the construction of a roof. Insulation is important and should be considered to retain as much heat in your sauna as possible. This is especially true in an outdoor free-standing sauna that cannot rely on the home's interior insulation.

BASEMENT SAUNA

Your sauna can also be built indoors wherever you have enough room. Many people decide to install their sauna in the basement because it offers the greatest amount of available space. A sauna doesn't require a great deal of space—as little as 9 square feet of floor—but many homes can't afford this space within the main living area. So to the basement it goes.

The overall idea is a room within a room (Fig. 7-10)—a controlled-atmosphere roomette with its own insulated walls, an insulated

door, and a self-contained heater. No special wiring is needed for smaller saunas, but you do have to match the heater to the size of the sauna. Remember to allow enough floor space for not only the heater but also for the wooden guard rail installed to prevent the bather from touching the hot metal accidentally.

Once you've insulated the framing members with 2½-inch-thick fiberglass, line the interior walls with either redwood or western red cedar tongue-and-grooved boards. The width of the boards must not exceed 6 inches, and sapwoods should be avoided where they may come in contact with your body. Why? Because they retain heat and can cause burns to your skin. Use heartwood.

CLOSET SAUNA

Have you decided against a sauna in your home because you think you don't have the space for it? Think again. If you can find a piece of free floor space three feet square, you can have

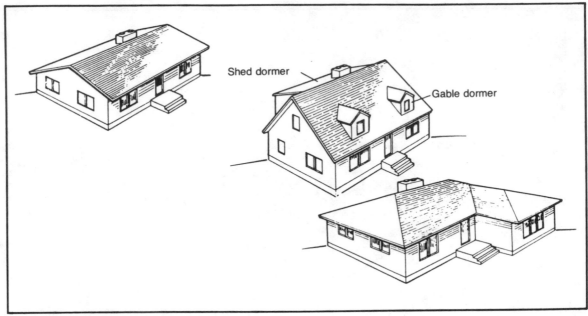

Fig. 7-4. Types of pitched roofs used in home construction.

your sauna. Just build a miniature room or line an existing closet, install a door, and you're all set. The door is the secret. Figure 7-11 illustrates the layout of a closet sauna while Fig. 7-12 shows the construction of the door. The 2-by-6-foot door has a heating unit, control, timer, window, and light fixture built in. It can be built or purchased with hinges and catches,

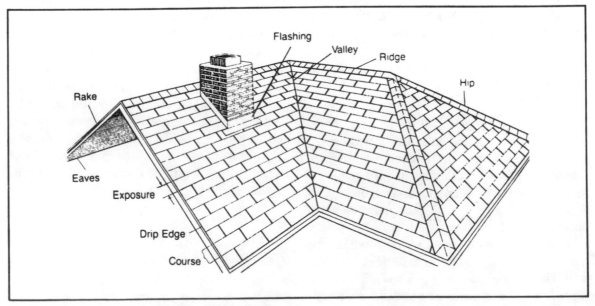

Fig. 7-5. Parts of typical roof. (Courtesy Georgia-Pacific)

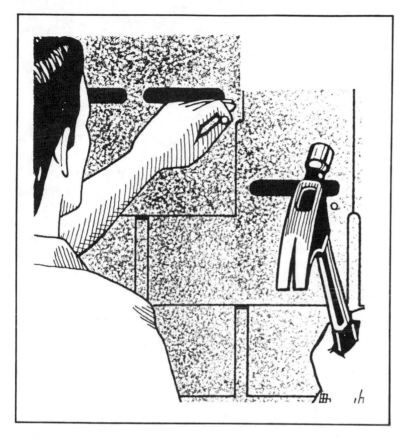

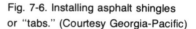

Fig. 7-6. Installing asphalt shingles or "tabs." (Courtesy Georgia-Pacific)

ready to connect to any ordinary 20-amp outlet. This type of a sauna door can be installed in a small closet near a bathroom for greatest efficiency.

BATHTUB SAUNA

You can even install a very simple version of the popular sauna in an enclosed bathtub. If you prefer long, warm soaks to short sessions in the dry heat of a sauna, you can install a radiant heat panel in the ceiling above an enclosed bathtub for a similar effect. It holds the temperature steady as it gives the effect similar to that of the sun's heat on the water. This is recommended for those who desire the benefits of a sauna, but cannot use one because of health limitations.

Your sauna can also be installed in the corner of a bathroom where it is both useful and convenient (Fig. 7-13).

THE SAUNA STOVE

The key component in every sauna is the heater or stove. For hundreds of years the sauna stove was heated with wood. Today's stoves are heated by oil, gas, or electricity, with a few wood sauna stoves still about (Fig. 7-14).

Your sauna stove dealer will help you in sizing your stove to coincide with the size and requirements of your sauna room or building. A typical sauna stove will cost from $300 to $600, with many models available above and below this range. Consider the need, placement, and installation of a vent pipe for your sauna. An indoor sauna may be able to be

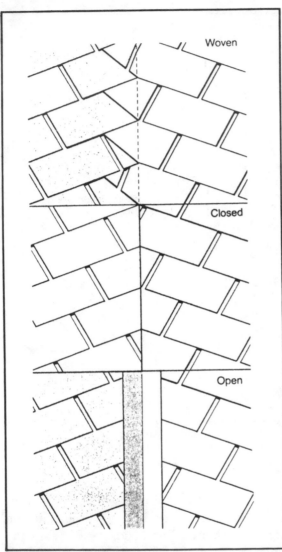

Fig. 7-7. Valley shingle application. (Courtesy Georgia-Pacific)

There are certain rules you must follow, however, to insure a healthful and safe sauna. Let's consider a few of the basic rules.

First, you should not smoke, exercise, or wear clothing in a sauna. It is to be a relaxing time without physical or mental stress.

Heat the sauna room to a temperature of 175 degrees Fahrenheit for about 30 minutes before entering it. Next, shower with soap and water to remove impurities and perspiration. Enter your sauna for 8 to 10 minutes, relaxing by sitting or laying on the bench. Then take a short, cold shower to close up your pores and invigorate your blood circulation. Re-enter the sauna for another 8 to 10 minutes of relaxation. Finally, take a long, cool shower to wash off perspiration and impurities from your skin

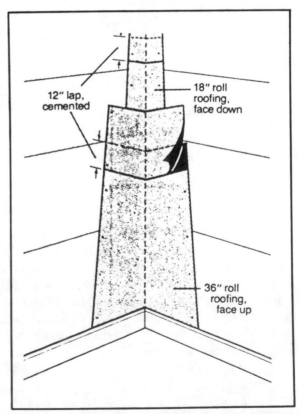

Fig. 7-8. Valley flashing installation. (Courtesy Georgia-Pacific)

vented to an existing flue or chimney—or may be limited to an electric unit needing no vent. You can vent your sauna stove either out the ceiling or through a nearby wall.

ENJOYING YOUR SAUNA

The sauna can be a very enjoyable part of your fitness center, offering physical and emotional toning to coincide with your exercise program.

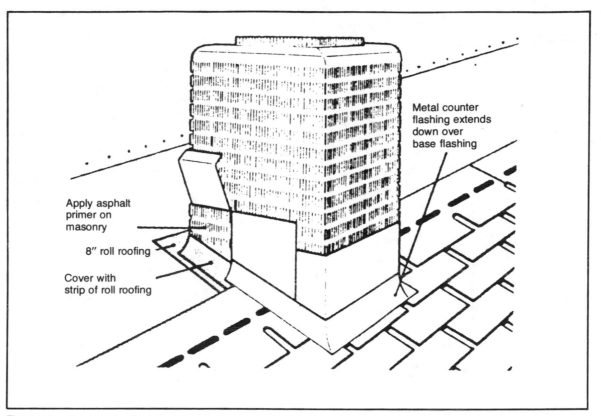

Metal counter flashing extends down over base flashing

Apply asphalt primer on masonry

8″ roll roofing

Cover with strip of roll roofing

Fig. 7-9. Installing roofing flashing. (Courtesy Georgia-Pacific)

while you encourage blood circulation. Now relax for 15 to 20 minutes before dressing.

There are other procedures for enjoying your sauna. Many will stay in longer for one session and follow it with a jump in the pool or spa. It's best to follow a sauna with a *cold* dunking because cold water will close up the pores of your skin and keep the impurities on the surface rather than allow them to re-enter your body. You want to wash them away as soon as your skin begins to cool. A cold water dunking is also very stimulating. In fact, those with heart conditions should discuss the effects with their doctor before planning, building, or using a traditional sauna.

To coincide with the installation and use of your sauna, let's consider the building of your own fitness bath.

Table 7-1. Estimating Roofing.

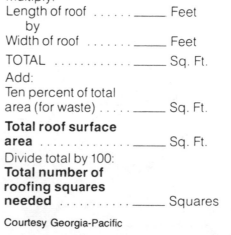

ESTIMATING FORM

Multiply:
Length of roof ...... _____ Feet
 by
Width of roof .... _____ Feet
TOTAL .... _____ Sq. Ft.
Add:
Ten percent of total
area (for waste) ..... _____ Sq. Ft.
**Total roof surface
area** .... _____ Sq. Ft.
Divide total by 100:
**Total number of
roofing squares
needed** .... _____ Squares

Courtesy Georgia-Pacific

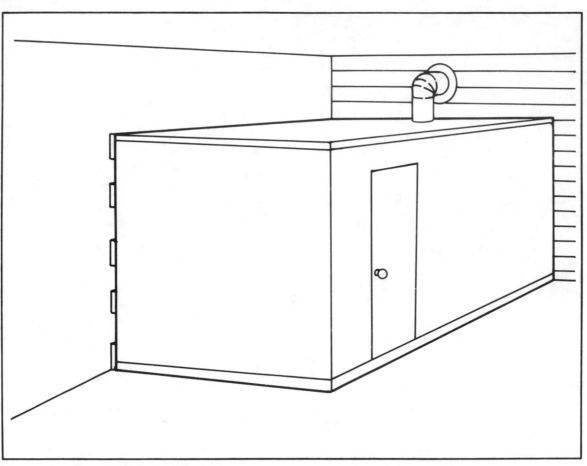

Fig. 7-10. Installing a sauna in your basement.

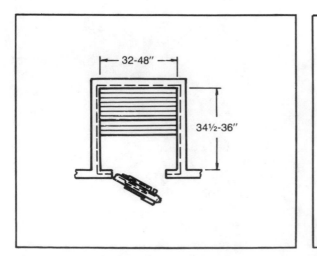

Fig. 7-11. Plan for building a sauna in your closet.

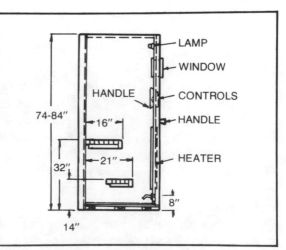

Fig. 7-12. Closet sauna door construction.

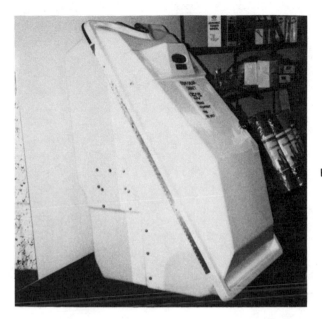

Fig. 7-13. Steam-sauna cabinet.

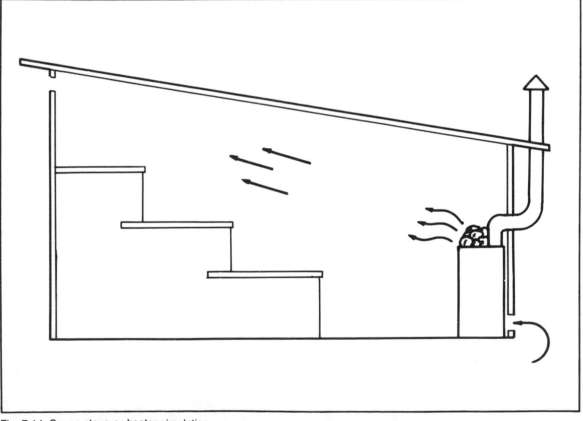

Fig. 7-14. Sauna stove or heater circulation.

8

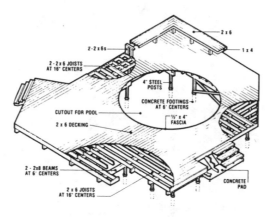

Fitness Bath

YOU'VE JUST FINISHED YOUR REGULAR WORK-out in your fitness center. Maybe you did an extra 20 chinups, two miles on the exercise bike, or one more press. You're perspiring and you're tired. What sounds best now is a dunk in a hot tub or spa, a shower, and maybe a session on the tanning bench. You're glad you decided to install a fitness bath (Fig. 8-1).

A *fitness bath* is a room that combines physical fitness equipment with water fitness: hot tub, spa, isolation tank, controlled environment room, whirlpool, or even an indoor swimming pool. A fitness bath is especially welcome at the end of a long workout or workday. It helps soothe you as it conditions your muscles.

Happily, a fitness bath can be added easily and often inexpensively by the do-it-yourselfer. In this chapter you'll learn the components of the fitness bath and how to construct and use them for greater enjoyment.

PLANNING

A fitness bath can save as many or as few elements as you desire. It can simply be a remodeled bathroom with an area for the storage and use of exercise equipment; or it can be as elaborate as a wetroom (Fig. 8-2). A well-stocked wetroom might include the following:

Spa. Eight-person oblong octagonal spa with transparent walls on five sides.

Tanning Bench. A 6-to-7-foot-long bench containing a series of ultraviolet tube lights. Some benches have an upper tier (like a waffle iron) so you can receive an even, all-over body tan without turning.

Shower Tier. Transparent enclosure and dressing area.

Isolation/Relaxation Tank. A tank in which heavily salinated water is heated to body skin temperature. When the tank is closed, you float in a prone position with no light, sound, or

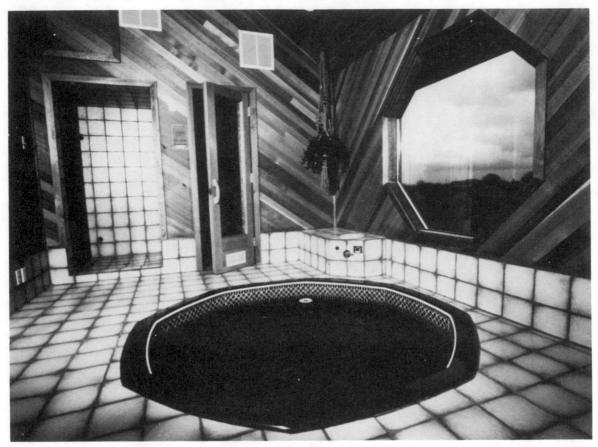

Fig. 8-1. Typical fitness bath with sauna, shower, and spa. (Courtesy National Spa and Pool Institute)

sensation of weight. Early research findings suggest that one hour of floating in the tank may prove promising as means to control tension headaches and enhance relaxation.

Controlled Environment Room. One room that fits two persons, seated. It acts as a sauna, steam room, shower, or tanning room, or any combination of these. Some rooms have adjustable lighting, stereo, and video.

Exercise Equipment Area. Any combination of indoor exercise equipment to suit your individual needs and desires.

Your fitness bath can also be remodeled from a garage, a garden, or an add-on. Figure 8-3 illustrates how an attached garden was

remodeled into a fitness bath using a hot tub with an entrance off the master bath. This fitness bath offers natural sunlight as well as privacy. To help you plan your fitness room, let's look specifically at the major elements, beginning with the spa or tub.

Although therapeutic heat and swirling waters pumped through hydrojets are similar in either a spa or hot tub, there are definite differences between the two. One difference is the air bubbler. In hot tubs, bubbles come from under and around the seats, whereas in most spas the bubbles come up directly through the floors and seats.

An authentic round hot tub is usually made with redwood. However, innovations now offer the buyer hot tubs in different shapes and woods, such as cedar, teak, oak, cypress, and mahogany. A spa is usually molded fiberglass with an inner acrylic or gelcoat finish. Spas of gunite or metal are less common, though they may be better for some sites. Forms and colors can be as free as your imagination.

For most people, the choice between the products is almost automatic because one or the other fits the purchaser better: a natural, rustic tub or a polished, sculptured spa.

THE HOT TUB

Hot tubs (Fig. 8-4) originated from old wood-

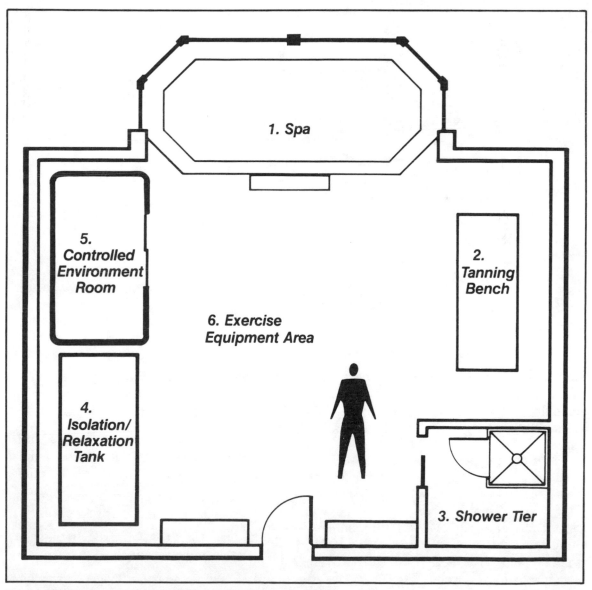

Fig. 8-2. Wetroom layout. (Courtesy National Spa and Pool Institute)

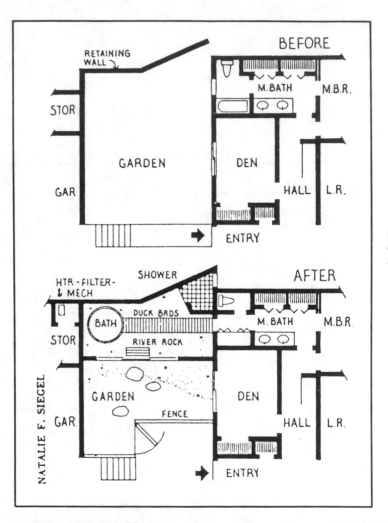

Fig. 8-3. Hot tub room addition—before and after. (Courtesy Western Wood Products Association)

en wine tanks. Even now, most tubs are still made just like wine casks, and often by the same firms. The constant soaking of the wood keeps tubs watertight without the use of single nail.

The most popular wood used in tub construction is redwood. Vertical grained, all-heart redwood is strong, watertight, aesthetically pleasing, and if properly maintained, will last for 15 years. Other trees with similarly durable and usable heartwoods include cedar, cypress, and oak. Teak is a well-proven, though expensive, wood. The main characteristics of the popular woods are:

☐ Redwood is extremely resistant to decay, does not splinter, and swells easily to watertightness.

☐ Cedar comes close to redwood on all counts, except it may not be as long-lived.

☐ Cypress is very durable and resistant to alkalis, acids, and other chemicals.

☐ Oak is a hardwood and extremely durable if well maintained.

☐ Teak is the unchallenged champion in durability and decay resistance. Also it has a natural oily smoothness. Price and availability are the drawbacks.

Typically tubs are 4 feet deep, but the range is anywhere from a uniform depth of 2½ feet to 5 feet. The most popular diameters are 5 and 6 feet. Widths can be scaled down to as little as 3½ feet or widened to as much as 12 feet or more. The standard 5 × 4 tub holds about 500 gallons of water and provides comfortable seating for four adults. The 6 × 4 tub holds 700 gallons of water and can comfortably seat five to six adults.

An average-sized redwood or cypress tub runs between $1,500 and $1,900 retail. Cedar tubs cost about $200 less. Oak, on the other hand, is almost double the redwood price in the same market. Teak is the most expensive of

them all, with prices depending largely on location and availability of the wood. With the additional cost of support equipment and installation, you can expect a wood hot tub to be between $3,800 and $5,300 in the current market.

It is possible to cut costs on the tub by choosing lesser cuts than heartwood, but you run the risk of splintering and water leaks. Some people save money by building their own hot tubs using kits and plans.

THE SPA

Traditionally, spas have been located next to swimming pools and constructed of cement or air-blown concrete. Today, the majority of contemporary spas are molded from multiple layers of fiberglass coated with acrylic or gel-

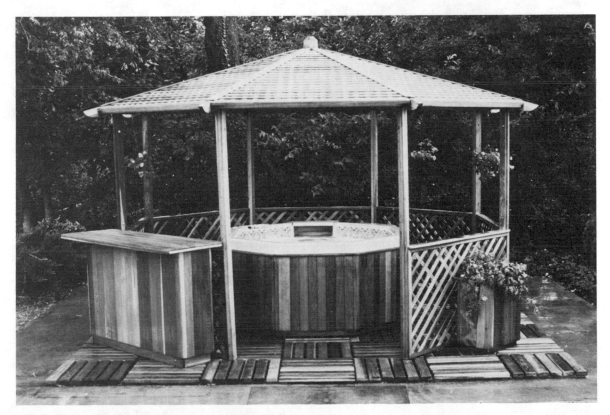

Fig. 8-4. Outdoor hot tub. (Courtesy National Spa and Pool Institute)

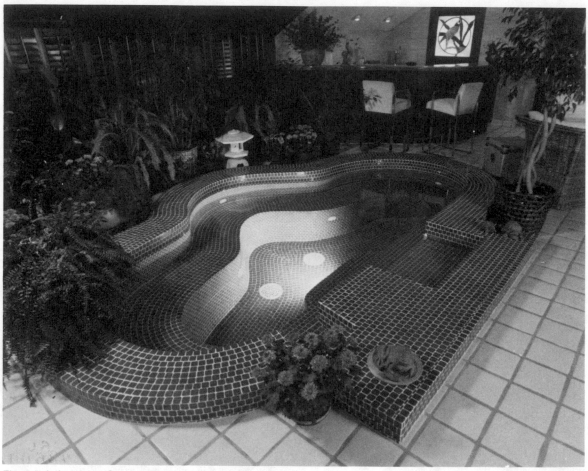

Fig. 8-5. Indoor spa. (Courtesy National Spa and Pool Institute)

coat. This combination allows one-piece construction in an almost infinite array of sizes, shapes, and colors. Fiberglass spas can be located inside or outside (Figs. 8-5 through 8-8), and the portable spa is a popular innovation. Fiberglass spas are easy to maintain and the smooth surface makes thorough cleaning a simple process. Leakage is not a concern.

A gelcoat fiberglass spa will cost you slightly less than an acrylic one, but gelcoat tends to be more susceptible to color fading and corrosion. Gelcoat generally requires more routine maintenance and often needs resurfacing after about five years.

Acrylic has become increasingly popular in spa manufacturing. Acrylic is thermoplastic which means it can be softened and formed by heat. The hard surface is very resistant to scratches and maintains its finish and color indefinitely.

Gelcoat and acrylic spas cost between $2,500 and $4,000 including support equipment. You can install it all yourself (Figs. 8-9 through 8-12) or add about 40 percent to the spa price for professional installation.

One of the more popular additions to the spa industry is the portable fiberglass spa. The electrical, heating, filtration, and pump equipment are all contained within the spa. It comes complete with an outer skin of wood or other material.

Although you can put a portable spa outdoors, most manufacturers make them simple to install indoors. The depth is limited so the spa can fit through a standard doorway. The energy source is a standard 110-volt outlet which should be on a separate circuit. Be sure the outlet is grounded and inspected by a licensed electrician.

Because portable spas are relatively new, they often are not Underwriter Laboratories' listed as a complete unit but as individual components. This does not mean they are unsafe, just that you should check each piece for the UL label.

The price of a portable spa is *lower* than all other types, ranging between $2,000 and $3,500 complete. Installation is usually nominal. And remember, one key purpose of a portable spa is for you to be able to take it with you. In our mobile society, a relocation or job change will always find you with your spa in tow.

SUPPORT EQUIPMENT

Once you've purchased your spa or hot tub,

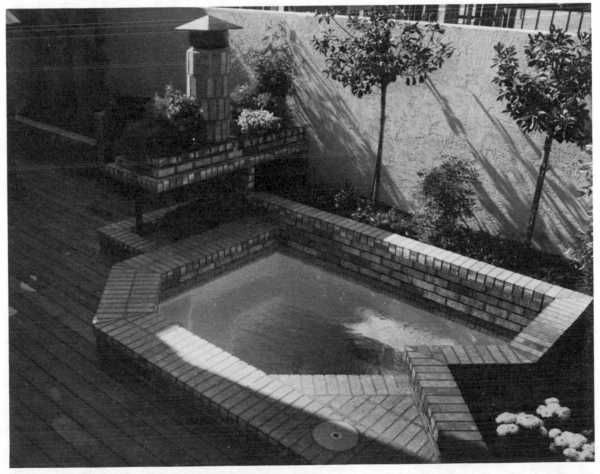

Fig. 8-6. Outdoor spa. (Courtesy National Spa and Pool Institute)

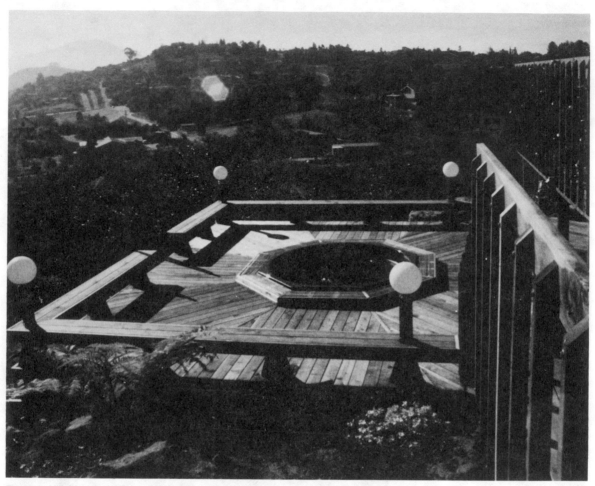

Fig. 8-7. Hillside spa built into deck. (Courtesy National Spa and Pool Institute)

you'll need support equipment to heat, circulate, and filter the water. Support equipment can be purchased separately or as a package, usually called a skid pack. It consists of pump, filter, heater, air blower, and necessary plumbing and hardware. The pump circulates water through the system. It usually powers hydrotherapy jets, commonly called hydrojets. The filter helps keep the water clean by removing minute particles of dirt, debris, and algae.

Whether you buy a skid pack or individual components, make sure all pieces are compatible, including your spa or tub. Let's look closer at each support equipment component.

Again, the pump circulates the water through the filter and heater in order to keep it clean and hot. The pump also powers the hydrojets in your spa or tub. When choosing a pump, important factors to consider are its capacity relative to the volume of water in your spa or hot tub, the number of hydrojets, the operating costs, and maintenance steps. Generally, a 1-horsepower (hp) motor is sufficient for a 500-gallon to 700-gallon spa or tub with four hydrojets.

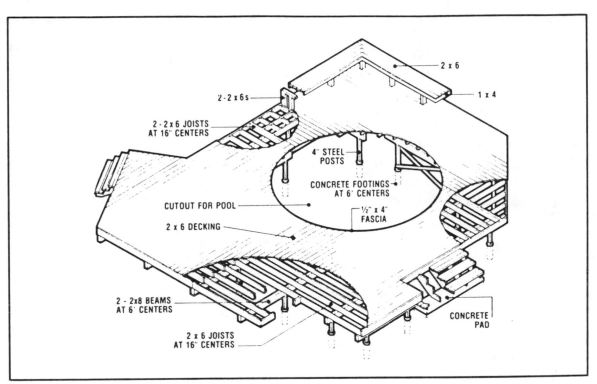

Fig. 8-8. Details for spa deck. (Courtesy Georgia-Pacific)

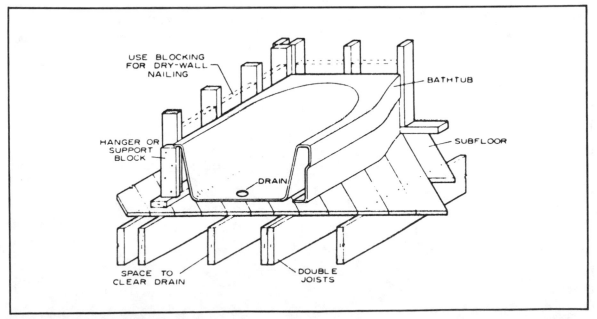

Fig. 8-9. Framing and installing a spa or tub.

155

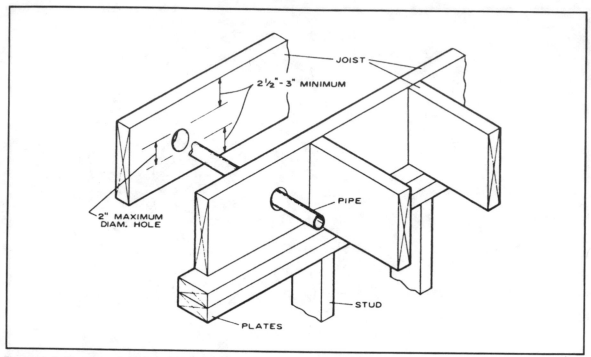

Fig. 8-10. Drilling through joists to install plumbing for spa or hot tub.

The filter's job is to keep the water fresh. There are different filter sizes, and the filter flow rate should be compatible with the pump.

There are generally three types of filters.

The cartridge filter, composed of nonwoven polyester, Dacron, or treated paper, traps dirt and residue as the water flows through it. A large majority of spas and tubs use cartridge

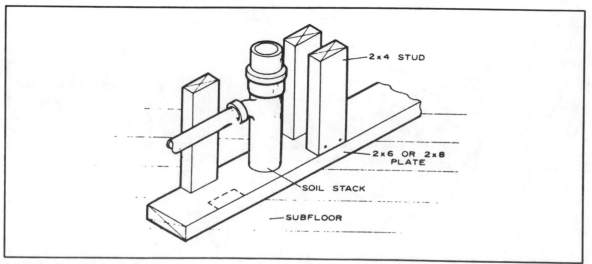

Fig. 8-11. Soil stack for plumbing.

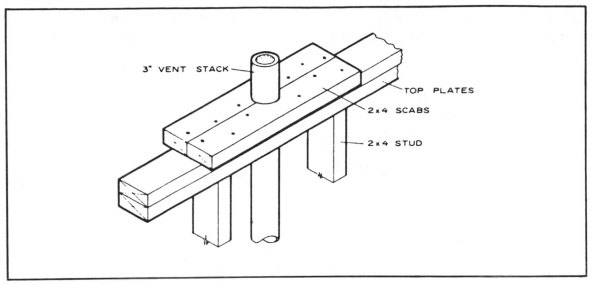

Fig. 8-12. Vent stack for plumbing.

filters. Properly maintained cartridges last one to two years before replacement is necessary. They do require regular cleaning with recommended cleaner more often, however.

For larger spas and hot tubs, DE (diatomaceous earth) filters are more efficient since they can carry a heavier dirt load than cartridge filters. Cleaning DE filters is more complicated than cartridge. When the DE filter needs to be cleaned, it must be backwashed (reverse-flow) or manually cleaned. A new coating of DE is applied, and then the filter is ready for its new cleaning cycle.

Sand filters operate similarly to the DE filter. They must be cleaned in a similar process, during which a portion of the water is lost. They offer a slightly less efficient filtration than DE.

Most heaters are either fossil-fueled (natural gas, propane, or heating oil) or electric. Your climate and type of vessel will help determine the most efficient energy source in your area. With natural gas, propane, and oil heaters, air and fuel are pulled into a burner and produce an open flame that heats copper

tubes or another heat transfer system. These heaters are designed to raise the water temperature quickly and may be more desirable in colder climates.

Electric heaters take longer to heat water but may be adequate for small installations, portable spas, or highly insulated spas. Electric heaters usually run continuously if the spa or tub is used often. Electric heaters make good backup systems for solar heaters. To date, the effectiveness of solar heaters for spas and tubs has yet to be proven. With the rapid advances in technology, however, solar heating might soon become a feasible alternative. Other alternatives include wood- and coal-burning heaters as well as heat exchangers.

Air blowers use small electric motors to produce thousands of tiny air bubbles. These motors must run at 15,000 to 22,000 rpm. Proper sizing and correct installation are the key factors for years of trouble-free performance. Little direct maintenance is required for the air blowers.

Powered by the pump, hydrojets produce aerated streams of water, creating a massage effect. Generally no maintenance is required except a thorough cleaning when you drain your spa or hot tub.

CHEMICALS

The chemistry of spa and hot tub water changes very quickly. Factors that cause this are high water temperatures, the aeration of the water, the body chemistry of the people using the spa or tub, and the high body-to-water ratio in the unit. For example, five people in a 500- to 700-gallon spa or tub equals about 250 people in an average size pool. The high water temperature also provides a good environment for algae and bacteria to grow. Because these factors change the water chemistry rapidly, water quality should be checked daily.

To keep your fitness bath's water fresh and clean, you need a water-quality test kit. They are easy to use and will give you the necessary information to keep the water clean and properly balanced. The kit should test the following:

☐ The chlorine/bromine disinfectant level.
☐ pH level.
☐ Total alkalinity.
☐ Calcium hardness.

Spa and hot tub water must have the correct balance of these elements. Unbalanced water can irritate eyes, corrode the equipment, and leave mineral deposits.

The most widely used chemicals for disinfecting spas or tubs are chlorine and bromine. Chlorine comes in liquid, tablet, or granulated forms. Bromine is available in sticks and tablets or a two-step dry chemical mixture. Both chemicals keep water free of harmful bacteria and prevent the growth of some algae when maintained at proper levels.

Potential hydrogen (pH) is the measurement of acidity or alkalinity (basicity) in the water. The scale runs from 0 to 14. The recommended pH range is 7.2 to 7.6. Below this, the water can corrode a spa or tub finish and support equipment; above this, the pH level can produce scaling, cloudy water or a clogged filter, and reduce the efficiency of the chlorine or, to a lesser degree, bromine.

Soda ash or sodium bicarbonate is used to raise pH level; muriatic acid or sodium bisulfate to lower it. As with any chemicals, carefully read and follow the directions for proper use of these substances.

Total alkalinity testing measures the amount of all alkaline salts in the water. Keep the total alkalinity in the recommended ranges of 90 to 150 parts per million (ppm). This will help you keep your pH level stable. It is also one good defense against forming excessive calcium carbonate, a type of alkalinity that causes scaling, cloudiness, and residue to form in your spa or tub.

Water should be tested for total alkalinity content every month. The same chemicals used to raise and lower pH are also used to control total alkalinity. Testing for water hardness is also important. Calcium is a mineral that affects the water's overall balance, and the ideal range is no more than 150 to 300 parts per million. If the calcium level is very high, it may be time to replace old water with new. If it is too low, add calcium chloride.

ACCESSORIES

A skimmer is perhaps the most necessary piece of "optional" equipment. Outdoors, it skims leaves and other contaminants off the surface of the water. Indoors, it skims perspiration and body oils from the water. The device prevents clogged drains and plumbing.

Some owners also supplement their filters with a water purification system. Such systems keep the water free from microorganisms by using purifying agents, like ozone or ultraviolet energy. Both these products, along with other purifying agents, are recognized as useful supplements to chlorine or bromine treatment.

Water purifying systems leave no residue in the water, remove most odors, and may even reduce the amounts of disinfectant required for proper water treatment. Most experts caution owners to use them only in addition to regular chemical purification, however. Chemical treatment of the water helps to kill microorganisms in still water or before they are pumped through the purifier.

Spa or hot-tub covers can be made out of fiberglass, canvas, plastic, or wood and are useful because:

□ They keep the water free of leaves and other objects when not in use.
□ They can act as a safety device to keep children out.
□ They keep heat in, thereby reducing energy costs.
□ They reduce the evaporation of water and chemicals.
□ They can be used as a winterizing cover.

If you've installed an indoor spa or tub in your fitness center, you can enjoy year-round hot soaks. Owners of outdoor models can soak year-round as well with some additional steps. A freeze-protection kit for your spa or tub includes:

□ Insulation for the unit, pipes, and support equipment.
□ Insulated cover to retain heat.
□ A device to protect your spa or tub from freezing that is mounted by a thermostat or time clock.

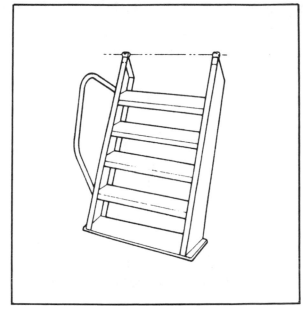

Fig. 8-13. Spa deck ladder. (Courtesy National Spa and Pool Institute)

If you close your spa or tub, carefully read the directions that come with your model and consult your dealer on the proper steps.

Other popular accessories, such as ladders (Figs. 8-13 through 8-15), inflatable pillows, trays, juice bars, toys, games, and back scrubbers can make your spa or hot tub an indoor or outdoor recreation and fitness center.

USING YOUR FITNESS BATH

For centuries, people have bathed in natural hot springs because of their supposed curative powers. Primitive cultures built temples around such springs, believing them to be the dwellings of gods and spirits. The Romans went a step further and built huge public baths for thousands of people. Today, hot mineral springs are still thought to have therapeutic value. Many famous resorts in the United States and Europe are based around natural mineral baths.

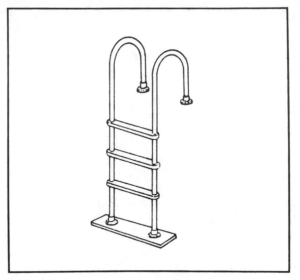

Fig. 8-14. In-pool ladder. (Courtesy National Spa and Pool Institute)

Modern professional athletes have also found value in a good, hot soak. Many professional sports teams prescribe hydrotherapy and hot tubs for players with painful joints and sore muscles. For the same reasons, a spa or hot tub is appreciated by anyone involved in a physical sport or activity. After a game of tennis or jogging, or even a hard day at the office, climbing into your jetted spa or hot tub is a good way to relax. A hot soak can relieve not only physical stress but mental stress and tension as well.

As one medical study put it, upon getting into warm bubbling water, "the first response to immersion at this temperature is a general and muscular relaxation. The hot water produces dilation of the blood vessels, or vasocilation, which is beneficial to the functioning of weak or spastic muscles and is usually sedative for those with chronic arthritis, muscle pains and neuralgia." In other words, it's easier for your heart to work, and muscle pain can be neutralized.

Other studies show that just being immersed in hot water slows down your pulse because your heart no longer has to fight against gravity. Your heart also enlarges slightly and works with 10 to 20 percent more efficiency. A hot soak improves blood flow to your entire body. Many other benefits are associated with hot water bathing, from relieving indigestion to helping you reduce body weight.

You can do stretching exercises that improve suppleness and flexibility and help to loosen tense muscles. When immersed in water to the neck, you weigh 90 percent less, so movement is easier and puts much less strain on your body. Spas and hot tubs also lend themselves to meditation techniques and other relaxation exercises.

As with any new piece of equipment, your spa or hot tub should be properly supervised for safe use. Persons with heart disease, diabetes, high or low blood pressure, and any serious illness, and pregnant women—indeed persons with any doubt—should not enter a spa or hot tub without prior consultation with their doctor.

There is a distinction between warm

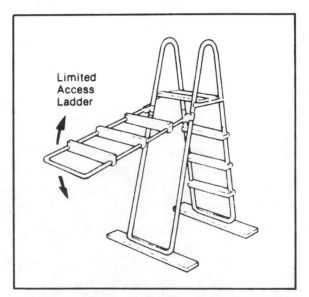

Fig. 8-15. Pool or spa limited access ladder. (Courtesy National Spa and Pool Institute)

water and hot—the maximum safe temperature is 104 degrees Fahrenheit (40 degrees Celsius). Fifteen minutes per soak is the recommended maximum time at this temperature.

WATER EXERCISES

If you have an indoor or outdoor swimming pool—or a large hot tub or spa—you can enjoy physical conditioning through water exercises. In the next few pages you'll discover fun fitness exercises you can do in a swimming pool or a large fitness bath.

During a workout the body should be warmed up by light conditioning and stretching exercises before heavier activities are attempted. Deck exercises including flexibility and strength activities with heavy breathing are appropriate. Various strokes may be simulated. Participants should begin with light rhythmical work at a slow pace. A tempo should be gradually accelerated, alternating slow with faster work, until you near perspiration. Through proper warm-up (Fig. 8-16), the body's deep muscle temperature will be raised and the ligaments and connecting tissues stretched. This prepares the body for vigorous work and helps avoid injury and discomfort.

Here is a regimen of high-potential physical activities which can be used in a small pool or in a limited area of a crowded institutional pool.

Alternate Toe Touch

Standing, in waste-to-chest-deep water, swimmer (Fig. 8-17):

1. Raises left leg bringing right hand toward left foot looking back and left hand extended rearward.
2. Recover to start position. Repeat. Reverse.

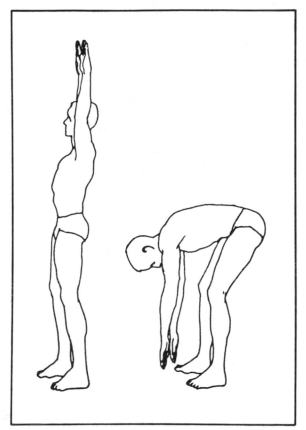

Fig. 8-16. Warming up to aquatic fitness.

Side Straddle Hop

Standing in waist-to-chest-deep water with hands on hips, swimmer (Fig. 8-18):

1. Jumps sideward to position with feet approximately two feet apart.
2. Recovers.

Toe Bounce

Standing in waist-to-chest-deep water with hands on hips, swimmer (Fig. 8-19):

1. Jumps high with feet together through a bouncing movement of the feet.
2. Repeat.

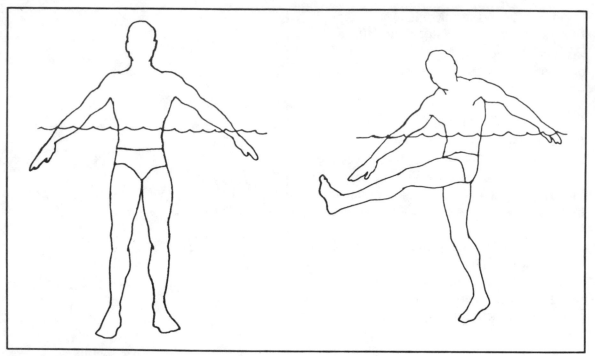

Fig. 8-17. Alternate toe touch.

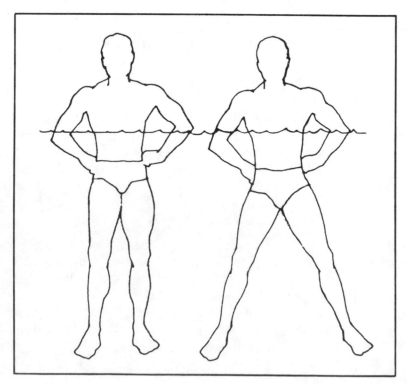

Fig. 8-18. Side straddle hop.

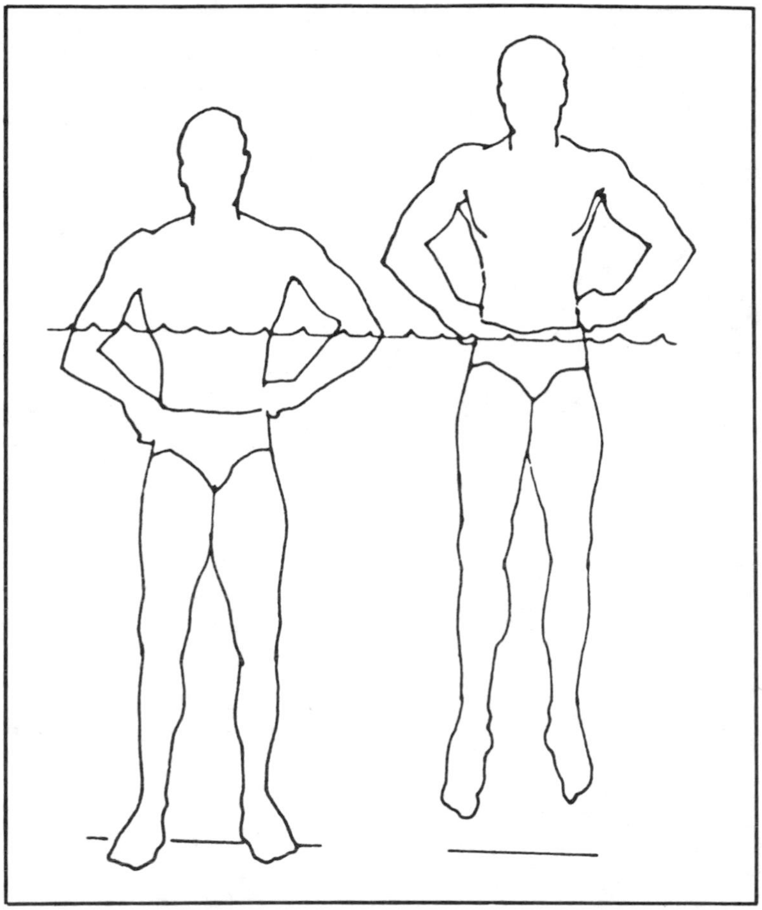

Fig. 8-19. Toe bounce.

Jogging in Place

Standing with arms bent in running position, swimmer (Fig. 8-20):

1. Jogs in place.

Leg Out

Standing at side of pool with back against wall, swimmer (Fig. 8-21):

1. Raises left knee to chest.
2. Extends left leg straight out.
3. Stretches leg.
4. Drops leg to starting position. Repeat. Reverse to right leg.

Pull and Stretch

Standing at side of pool with back against wall, swimmer (Fig. 8-22):

1. Raises left leg and clasps calf with both arms pulling leg vigorously to the chest.
2. Recovers to starting position.
3. Raises right leg and clasps calf with both arms pulling leg vigorously to the chest.
4. Recovers to the starting position.

Poolside Knees Up

Supine, holding on to pool gutter with hands

163

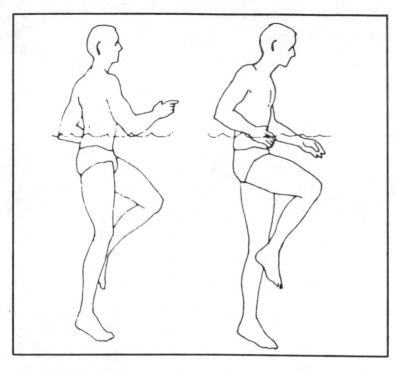

Fig. 8-20. Jogging in place.

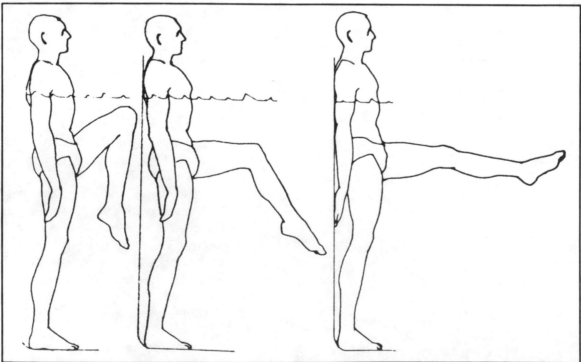

Fig. 8-21. Leg-out aquatic fitness exercise.

164

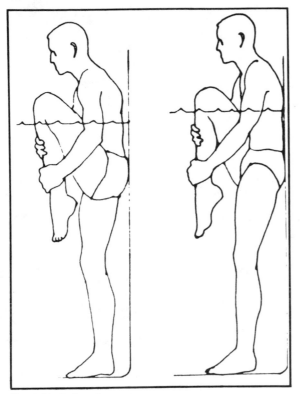
Fig. 8-22. Pull and stretch.

and legs extended, swimmer (Fig. 8-23):

1. Brings knees to chin.
2. Recovers to the starting position. Repeat.

Raising Hips

Prone, holding on to pool gutter with one hand flat on wall to push legs out, swimmer (Fig. 8-24):

1. Raises hips, holding for four counts.
2. Relaxes. Repeat.

Leg Swing Outward

Standing with back against poolside, and hands sideward holding gutter, swimmer (Fig. 8-25):

1. Raises left foot as high as possible with leg straight.
2. Swings foot and leg to left side.

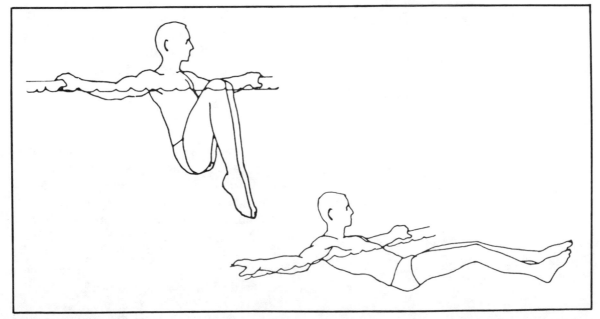
Fig. 8-23. Poolside knee up.

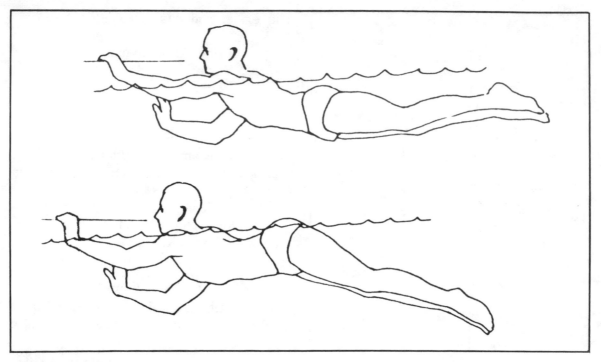

Fig. 8-24. Raising hips.

3. Recovers to starting position by pulling left leg vigorously to right. Repeat. Reverses to right leg. Repeat.

Climbing

Hands in pool gutter, facing poolside and feet flat against side and approximately 16 inches apart, swimmer (Fig. 8-26):

1. Walks up side by approximately six short steps.
2. Walks down side to starting position. Repeat.

Elementary Bobbing

Standing in shallow water, swimmer (Fig. 8-27):

1. Takes a breath.

2. Submerges in a tuck position with feet on the pool bottom in shallow water. Exhales during (2) and (3).
3. Shoves up off bottom and regains a standing position.
4. Inhales with head out of water.
5. Repeat (2), (3), and (4), etc.

HAVING FUN

As you can see, your fitness bath can be both relaxing and invigorating as you exercise in the water. You'll also gain exercise as you build and or install your own fitness bath.

Information on how to plumb your fitness bath can be found in *The Complete Handbook of Plumbing* by Robert E. Morgan (TAB book No. 1374). How-to-do-it information on how to install a deck for your spa, hot tub, or pool is offered in *The Complete Book of Fences* by Dan Ramsey (TAB book No. 1508).

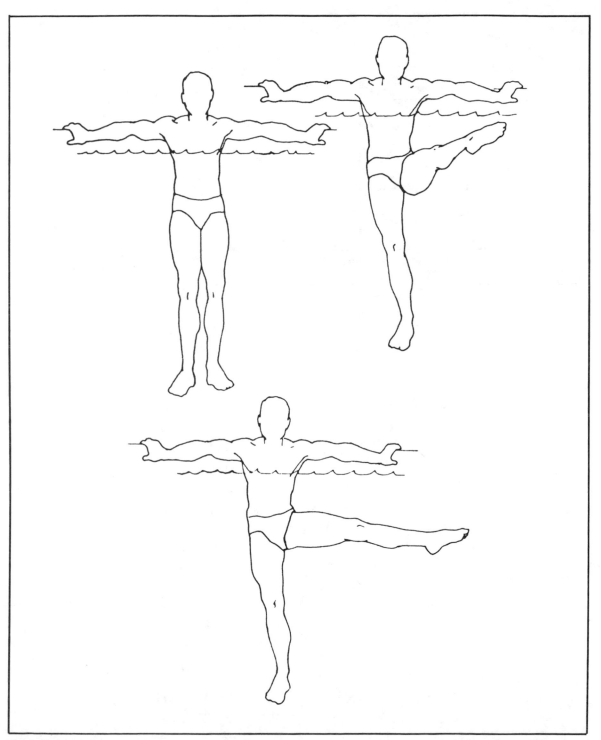

Fig. 8-25. Leg swing outward.

167

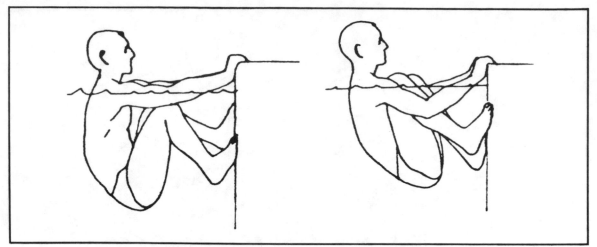

Fig. 8-26. Climbing exercise for your pool or fitness bath.

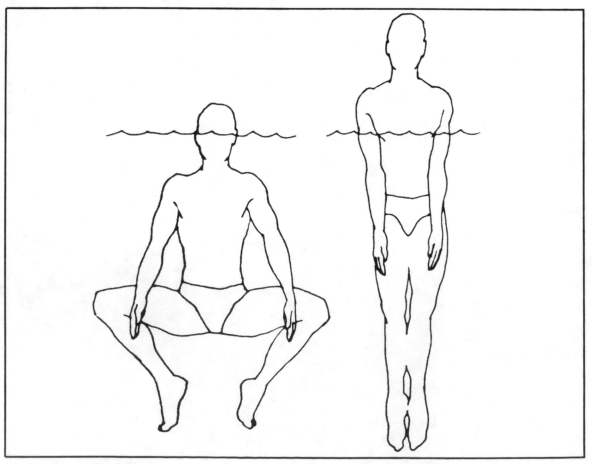

Fig. 8-27. Elementary bobbing.

168

9

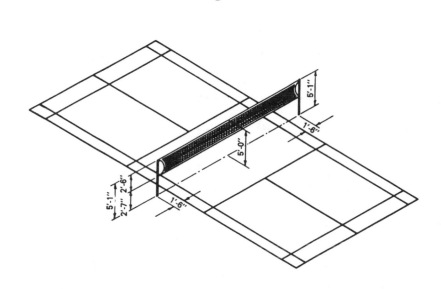

Outdoor Fitness Center

THERE ARE MANY GOOD REASONS WHY YOU should consider building part or all of your fitness center outdoors.

First, the great outdoors offers more space. Your living quarters may already be cramped, and the addition of even an exercise bike may require a major replanning of traffic patterns and furniture locations. Outdoors you can install courts and equipment without worrying about walls and other hindrances.

Second, during most seasons and in many parts of the country, it's more healthful to work out outdoors. You gain the healthful benefit of having fresh air to breath as you inhale. Of course, in some large cities, you may want to move your exercises *indoors* for the same reasons: the air.

Another reason for outdoor fitness it that there are many activities that are difficult if not impossible to duplicate indoors—unless you live in the Superdome! You may find greatest recreation in playing baseball, soccer, football, tennis, golf, track, or similar games.

So the purpose of this chapter is to guide you in the selection, installation, and use of outdoor fitness facilities. Don't be intimidated by the size of these fields and facilities. In most cases, they can be as easy to install as indoor fitness equipment. Let's take a look at the requirements for the more popular fitness facilities before considering simple construction methods.

TENNIS COURT

Tennis is still one of the most popular outdoor fitness games for the amateur athlete. It offers the development of coordination skills while teaching sportsmanship and offering recreation.

Figure 9-1 illustrates the layout of a tennis court as suggested by the United States Lawn Tennis Association. You'll need a

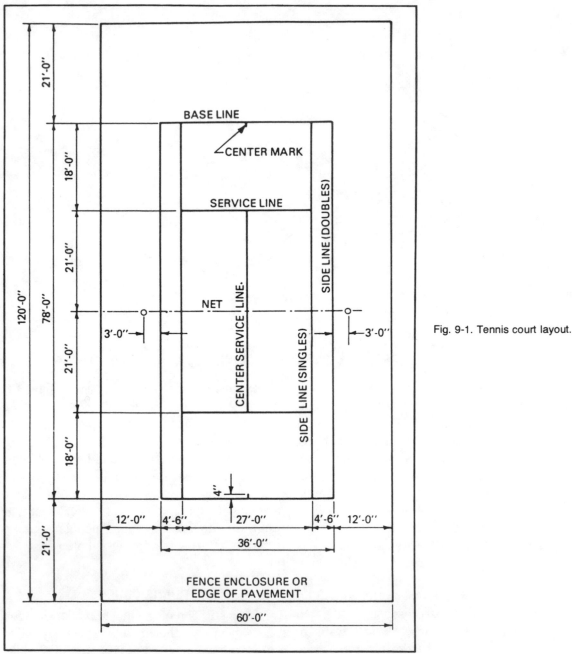

Fig. 9-1. Tennis court layout.

minimum of 7200 square feet of ground space to install this court, but you can do it in less if you need to. The playing court is 36 feet by 78 feet, plus at least 12 feet clearance on both sides or between courts in battery and 21 feet clearance on each end. The best orientation of the long axis should be north-south so that the sun doesn't interfere with play as much.

The tennis court surface may be concrete, or bituminous material with specialized protective colorcoating, or sand clay. Drainage may be from end to end, side to side, or corner to corner diagonally at a minimum slope of 1 inch in 10 feet for pavement and level for sand clay with underdrainage.

A fence is often installed around a tennis court to a height of up to 10 feet. General fence installation details will be offered later in this chapter.

All measurements for court markings are to the outside of lines, except for those involving the center service line which is equally divided between the right and left service courts. Court markings should be 2 inches wide. Figure 9-2 offers an isometric drawing showing the dimensions and placement of the tennis court net.

BADMINTON

Badminton is another popular court game that can be a source of fun as well as fitness. Figure 9-3 shows the layout for a badminton court as suggested by the American Badminton Association. Ground space needed is 1620 square feet to the edge of the pavement. A single court is 17 feet by 44 feet, and doubles court is 20 feet by 44 feet with a 5-foot minimum unobstructed area on all sides. As with the tennis court, preferred orientation is for the long axis to be north-south.

Court surface should be concrete or bituminous material with optional protective colorcoating for permanent installation. Badminton may be played on a turf court for general recreation use. All court markings should be 1½ inches wide and preferably white or yellow in color. Figure 9-4 offers an isometric drawing of the badminton net layout.

VOLLEYBALL

In between the large tennis court and the smaller badminton court is the volleyball

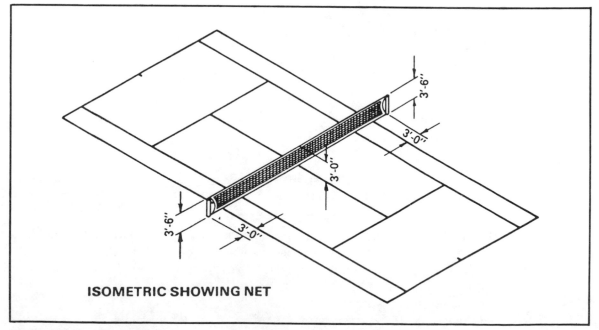

ISOMETRIC SHOWING NET

Fig. 9-2. Tennis court net layout.

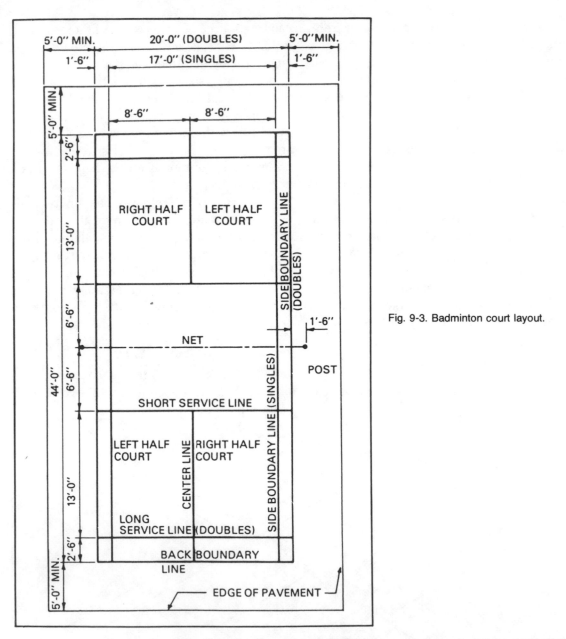

5'-0" MIN. 20'-0" (DOUBLES) 5'-0" MIN.

1'-6" 17'-0" (SINGLES) 1'-6"

5'-0" MIN.

8'-6" 8'-6"

2'-6"

RIGHT HALF COURT LEFT HALF COURT

SIDE BOUNDARY LINE (DOUBLES)

13'-0"

6'-6"

1'-6"

44'-0"

NET

POST

6'-6"

SHORT SERVICE LINE

SIDE BOUNDARY LINE (SINGLES)

LEFT HALF COURT RIGHT HALF COURT

CENTER LINE

13'-0"

SIDE BOUNDARY LINE (DOUBLES)

LONG SERVICE LINE (DOUBLES)

2'-6"

BACK BOUNDARY LINE

5'-0" MIN.

EDGE OF PAVEMENT

Fig. 9-3. Badminton court layout.

court, requiring about 4000 square feet of ground space. Figure 9-5 depicts a volleyball court layout from the United States Volleyball Association. Playing court is 30 feet by 60 feet plus 6 to 10 feet unobstructed space on all sides. Surface, drainage, and orientation are all suggested as those for the tennis court and badminton court. Court markings should be 2 inches wide except as noted. Figure 9-6 illustrates the layout for the volleyball net.

BASKETBALL

Few games are more American than basket-

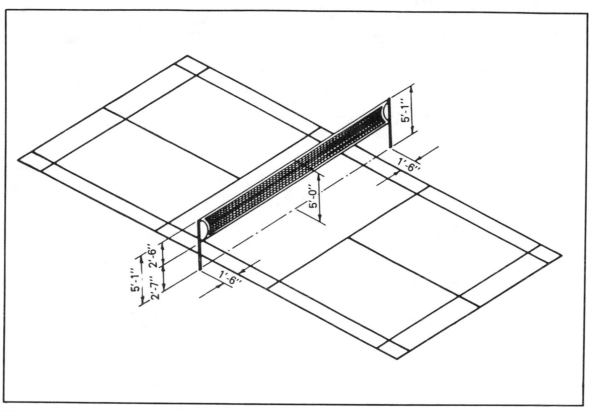

Fig. 9-4. Badminton court net layout.

ball. It is also one of the most popular with amateur athletes and is played in many driveways.

Figure 9-7 shows the layout of a basketball court as suggested by the Amateur Athletic Union. The court is about 46 by 85 feet. Figure 9-8 shows the layout and construction of a rectangular backboard. The backboard can be constructed of any rigid weather-resistant material, painted white. Lines on the court should be 2 inches wide.

BASEBALL

Figure 9-9 illustrates the diamond layout for Babe Ruth and Senior League Baseball. You'll need about 3 acres of ground for this ballpark. Baselines are 90 feet. Pitching distance is 60 feet 6 inches. The pitcher's plate is 10 inches

above the level of home plate. Distance down foul lines is 320 feet to 350 feet. Outfield distance to center field is 400 feet. For Senior League Baseball, recommended distance from home plate to all outfield fence points is 300 feet or more.

Optimum orientation is to locate home plate so that the pitcher is throwing across the sun and the batter is not facing it. The line from home plate through the pitcher's mound and second base should run east-northeast. A backstop should be installed from 40 to 60 feet behind home plate. Of course, these are all the "official" numbers. You can build your own baseball diamond to any size you desire.

The playing surface should be turf. The infield may be skinned and should be graded so that the base lines and home plate are level.

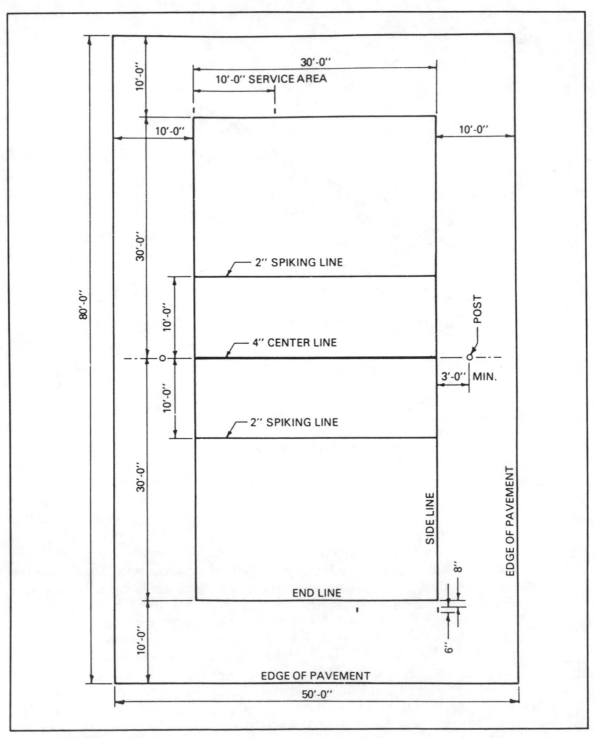

Fig. 9-5. Volleyball court layout.

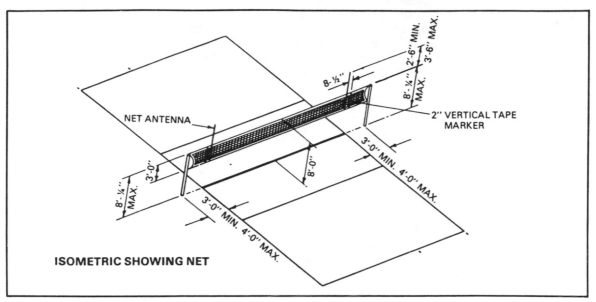

ISOMETRIC SHOWING NET

Fig. 9-6. Volleyball court net layout.

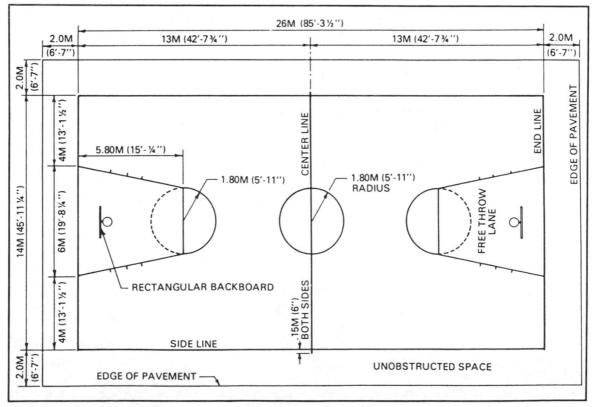

Fig. 9-7. AAU basketball court layout.

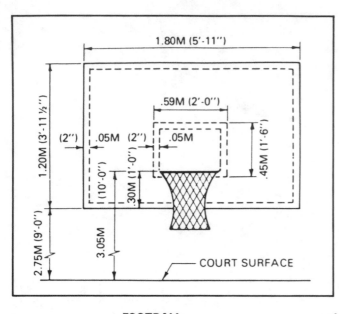

Fig. 9-8. AAU rectangular backboard layout.

FOOTBALL

Figure 9-10 offers the layout for an 11-man football field as suggested by the National Collegiate Athletic Association (NCAA). Ground space is 64,000 square feet, or about 1½ acres. Playing field width is 160 feet and length is 360 feet. You'll also want a minimum of 6 feet on all sides of unobstructed space. Preferred orientation is for the long axis to be northwest-southeast to suit the angle of the sun in the fall playing season, or north-south for longer periods. The surface should be turf. Figure 9-11 shows construction details for goal posts.

SOCCER

There's been increased interest in soccer during the past decade with soccer fields and teams popping up across the country. Figure 9-12 offers the playing field layout for men's and boys' soccer, as suggested by the NCAA. Recommended area is 1.7 acres to 2.1 acres. Playing field width is 195 to 225 feet with length proposed at 330 to 360 feet. Preferred orientation is for the long axis to be

northwest-southeast to suit the angle of the sun in the fall playing season, or north-south for longer periods. Figure 9-13 shows the construction of soccer goal posts.

GOLF DRIVING RANGE

Golf is still a very popular sport for developing fitness and fun. While most people don't have the room to construct their own golf course, many can find room for a golf driving range in their backyard or nearby vacant lots.

To guide you in designing your own golf driving range, Fig. 9-14 illustrates a "regulation" range with 25 tees as suggested by the National Golf Federation. You will need only one or two and a 300-yard range length may be ambitious.

RUNNING TRACK

You probably don't have enough room to install your own quarter mile running track (Fig. 9-15), but you may be able to use this plan to mark out a track on a nearby vacant lot, power-line right-of-way, or playing field. The 276 feet

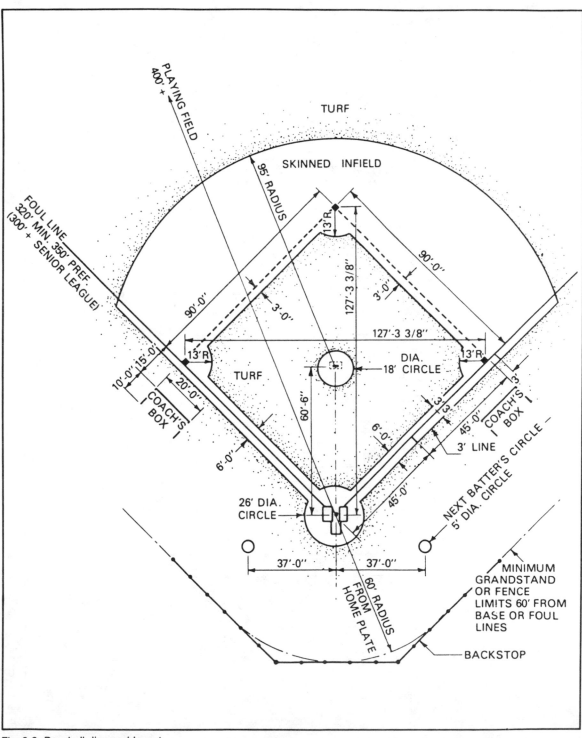

Fig. 9-9. Baseball diamond layout.

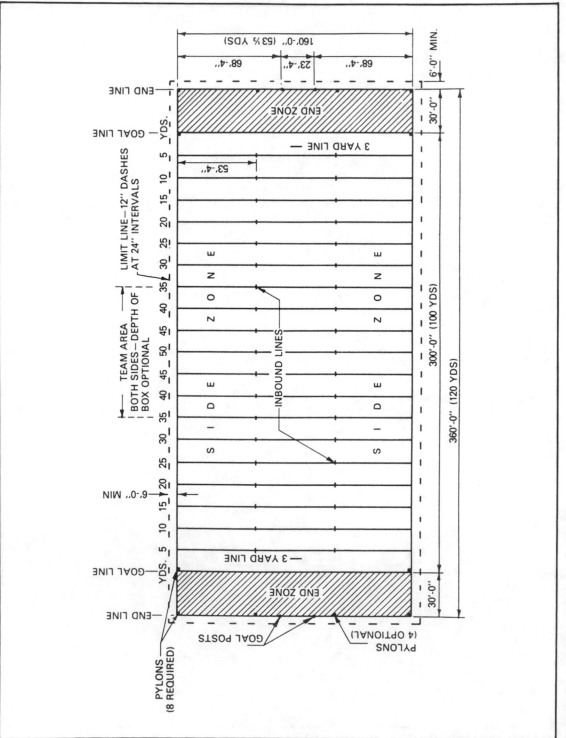

Fig. 9-10. Eleven-man football playing field layout.

178

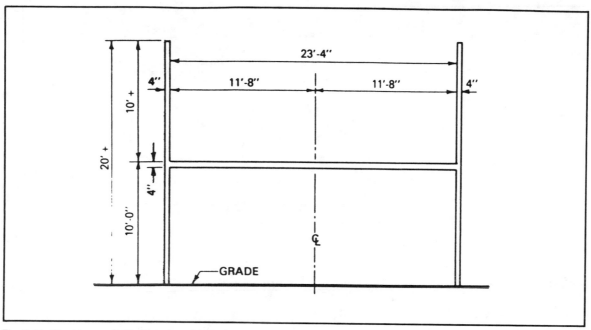

Fig. 9-11. Eleven-man football goal post layout.

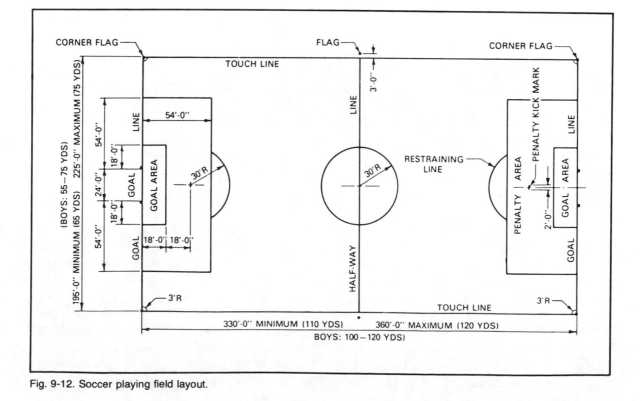

Fig. 9-12. Soccer playing field layout.

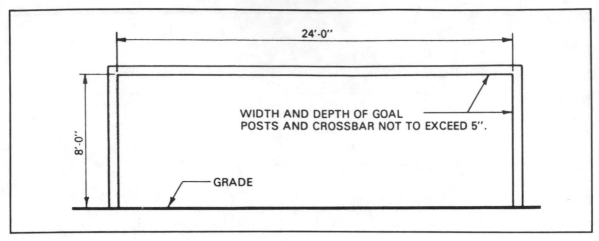

Fig. 9-13. Soccer goal post detail.

by 600 feet layout will give you a quarter-mile run per revolution. Ground space is about 4.3 acres. The track should be oriented so that the long axis falls in a sector from north-south to northwest-southeast with the finish line at the northerly end.

HORSESHOE COURT

Here's one fitness sport that can be laid out in many backyards: a horseshoe court. Figure 9-16 shows such a court as suggested by the National Horseshoe Pitchers' Association of America. Ground space needed is 1400 square feet, including clear space. The playing court is 10 by 50 feet plus a recommended 10-foot minimum unobstructed area on each end and a 5-foot minimum wide zone on each side. Recommended orientation is for the long axis to be north-south.

Surface of the playing area, except for boxes and optional walkways, should be turf. Area should be pitched to the side at a maximum slope of 2 percent. Elevation and slant of steel pegs should be between 2 and 3 inches and equal. The boxes are to be filled with gummy potter's or blue clay for competition. A 2-foot high backstop should be con-

structed at the end of the box to intercept overthrown or bounding shoes.

ARCHERY TARGET RANGE

Figure 9-17 offers the layout for an archery range as suggested by the National Archery Association. Again, it can be modified for non-competition practice at home based on your skills and space.

Figure 9-18 illustrates the construction of the actual archery target. Target papers can be purchased through sporting good stores. It is very important that a buffer zone or backstop be available behind the targets for overshot arrows to eliminate damage or injury.

FENCES

Now that you've seen how larger outdoor fitness facilities are laid out, let's look at construction details for fences, nets and posts, playing surfaces, and backstops.

Figure 9-19 is an elevation of a typical fence that can be used to contain outdoor fitness centers. Fence posts are typically a minimum of schedule 40 weight with the chain link fabric galvanized coating per ASTM A392 or ASTM A491. Top and bottom selvage

180

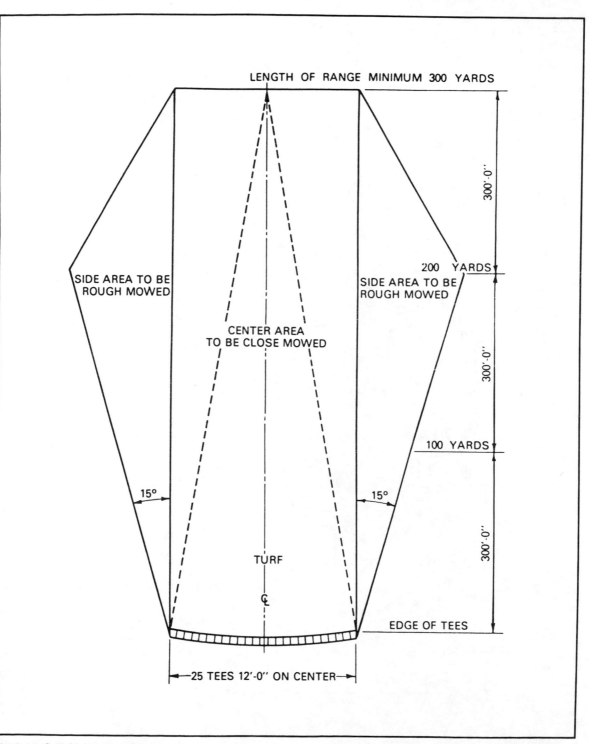

Fig. 9-14. Golf driving range layout.

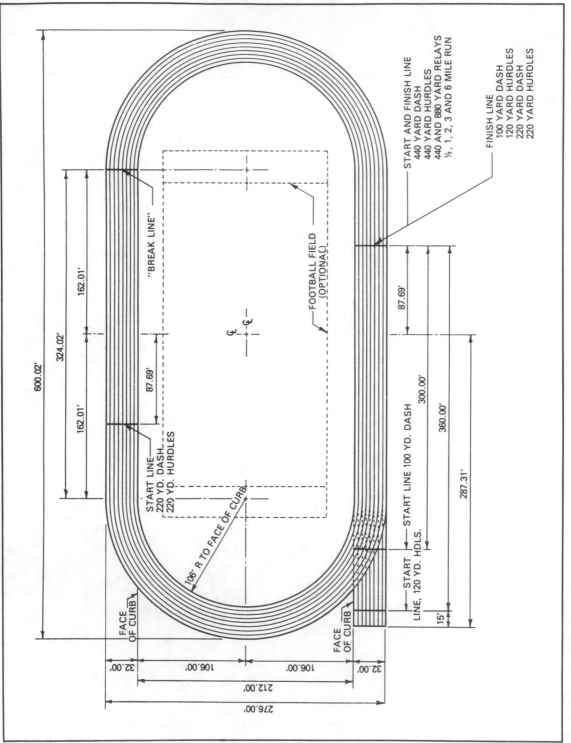

Fig. 9-15. Layout of ¼-mile running track.

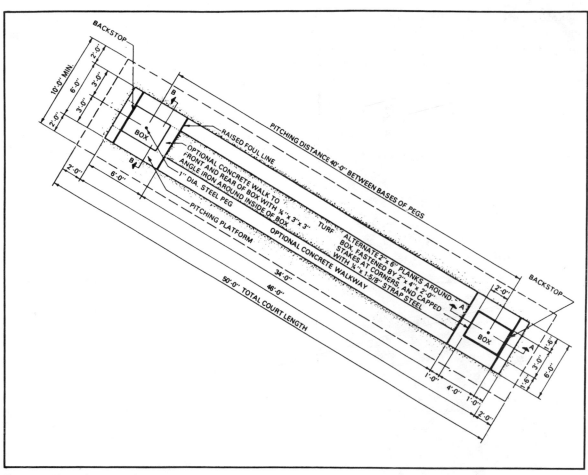

Fig. 9-16. Horseshoe court layout.

should be knuckled. Gates should have offset hinges and a latching device that allows access to a padlocking device from both sides.

Additional information on the construction and installation of all types of fences can be found in my book *The Complete Book of Fences* (TAB book No. 1508).

POSTS

Posts are installed to support tennis, badminton, and other nets. A typical illustration is Fig. 9-20 showing a tennis net and post details.

Post pipes should be 2⅞ inches (outside diameter) for badminton, paddle tennis, plat-

form tennis, and tennis; volleyball post pipes should be 3½ inches outside diameter. Footings should be of concrete, with a 16-inch minimum diameter for end posts and a depth of 4 feet or to the frost line. The top of the concrete should slope away from the post.

Sometimes it's more practical to install removable posts so that equipment can be taken away when not in use to make way for other activities. Figure 9-21 illustrates the construction of a removable post.

BACKSTOPS

For safety of spectators and nearby buildings,

backstops are often constructed behind home plate at softball and baseball fields. Figure 9-22 shows the installation of a regulation softball backstop. Figure 9-23 offers the layout of a regulation baseball backstop.

Posts for backstop heights up to 16 feet should be 3 inches (O.D.). Posts for backstop heights 18 to 24 feet should be 4 inches (O.D.). Top, intermediate, and bottom rails can be of 1⅝-inch pipe.

PLAYING SURFACES

We've talked about playing surfaces a few times in discussing the construction of playing fields and outdoor fitness centers. Figure 9-24 shows the installation of four popular sports playing surfaces: natural turf, concrete paving, sand clay, and bituminous concrete.

On installing natural turf, subgrade to pitch in the same direction as the surface and slope to underdrains. Filter course, 4 to 6 inches, is to be used only when subsoil conditions require. There should be a minimum of 6 inches of top soil or 8 inches of prepared soil.

Concrete paving should be reinforced in 6-inch-by-6-inch squares with #6 gauge welded wire fabric. Minimum thickness is 4 inches. Expansion joints are installed as needed.

There are three courses to laying sand

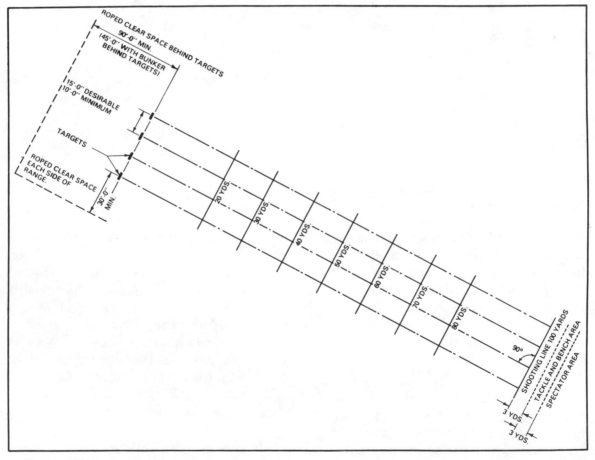

Fig. 9-17. Archery range layout.

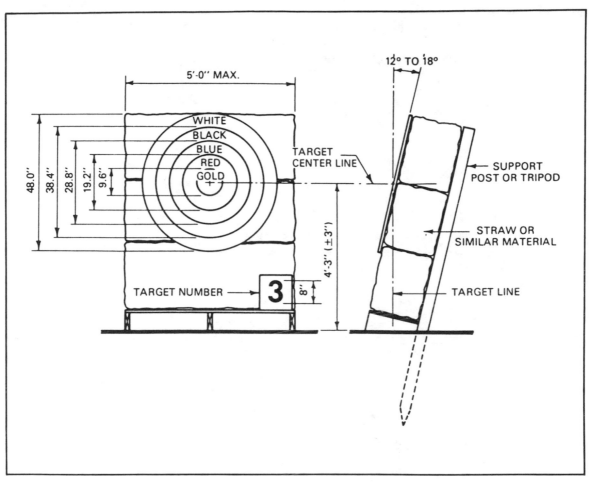

Fig. 9-18. Archery target details.

clay. The filter course of 4 to 6 inches may be omitted if local soil conditions are suitable. Base course should be a minimum of 3 inches of crushed stone and crushed fines. The surface course is a minimum of 4 inches in two lifts.

Bituminous material should have a 4-inch base course over a minimum 6-inch filter course. The surface should be at least 2½ inches in two lifts. A sealcoat can be applied on a smooth asphalt surface at the manufacturer's recommended rate.

Figures 9-25 through 9-31 and Tables 9-1 and 9-2 offer construction plans for an outdoor fitness center storage unit.

MOVING THE INDOORS OUTDOORS

In addition to these larger fitness fields and facilities, nearly any of the indoor fitness equipment covered in earlier chapters of this book can be moved outdoors—provided the weather is cooperative. In fact, many people intentionally retain the portability of smaller fitness equipment so that they can enjoy perspiring in the sun.

Remember, though, that fitness equipment made of wood should be treated before installation. Metal should be chromed or galvanized. You may wish to make some or all of

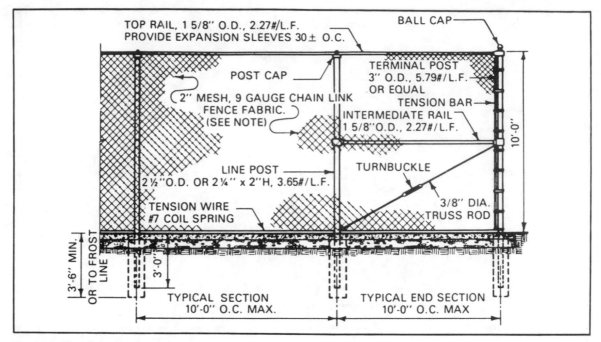

TOP RAIL, 1 5/8" O.D., 2.27#/L.F.
PROVIDE EXPANSION SLEEVES 30 ± O.C.

BALL CAP

POST CAP

2" MESH, 9 GAUGE CHAIN LINK
FENCE FABRIC.
(SEE NOTE)

TERMINAL POST
3" O.D., 5.79#/L.F.
OR EQUAL

TENSION BAR

INTERMEDIATE RAIL
1 5/8"O.D., 2.27#/L.F.

LINE POST
2½"O.D. OR 2¼" x 2"H, 3.65#/L.F.

TURNBUCKLE

TENSION WIRE
#7 COIL SPRING

3/8" DIA.
TRUSS ROD

10'-0"

3'-6" MIN.
OR TO FROST LINE

3'-0"

TYPICAL SECTION
10'-0" O.C. MAX.

TYPICAL END SECTION
10'-0" O.C. MAX

Fig. 9-19. Elevation of typical outdoor court fence.

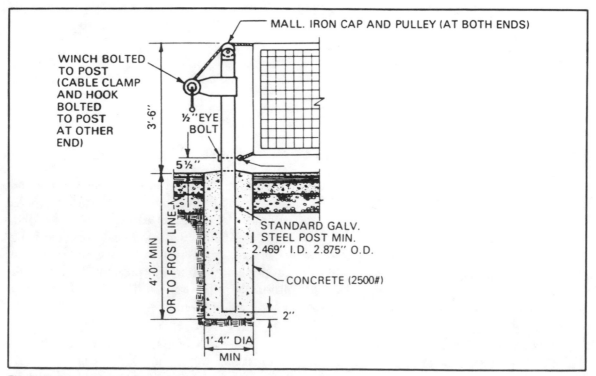

MALL. IRON CAP AND PULLEY (AT BOTH ENDS)

WINCH BOLTED
TO POST
(CABLE CLAMP
AND HOOK
BOLTED
TO POST
AT OTHER
END)

½"EYE
BOLT

3'-6"

5½"

4'-0" MIN
OR TO FROST LINE

STANDARD GALV.
STEEL POST MIN.
2.469" I.D. 2.875" O.D.

CONCRETE (2500#)

2"

1'-4" DIA
MIN

Fig. 9-20. Tennis net and post details.

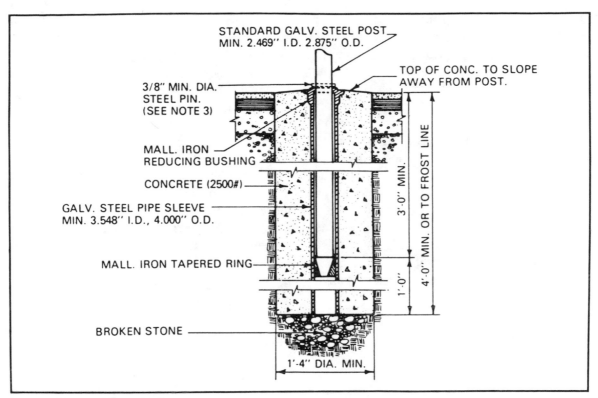

STANDARD GALV. STEEL POST
MIN. 2.469" I.D. 2.875" O.D.

TOP OF CONC. TO SLOPE
AWAY FROM POST.

3/8" MIN. DIA.
STEEL PIN.
(SEE NOTE 3)

MALL. IRON
REDUCING BUSHING

CONCRETE (2500#)

GALV. STEEL PIPE SLEEVE
MIN. 3.548" I.D., 4.000" O.D.

MALL. IRON TAPERED RING

BROKEN STONE

3'-0" MIN.

4'-0" MIN. OR TO FROST LINE

1'-0"

1'-4" DIA. MIN.

Fig. 9-21. Removable post details.

your fitness equipment portable so that you can move it indoors or out-of-doors easily to take advantage of seasons and weather.

YOUR JOGGING COURSE

Jogging is a form of exercise that consists either of alternate walking and running at a slow-to-moderate pace or running at a slow steady pace. The amount of intensity of exercise performed while jogging may be varied over a wide range by regulating the total distance covered, the ratio of walking to running, and the pace of running.

Jogging is of particular value since it provides the opportunity for a graduated program of physical activity that can be performed by most people regardless of age, sex, or level of physical fitness. It doesn't require much in the

way of special skills, equipment, facilities, or supervision, nor does it require locating teammates or opponents as do many sports or games. Jogging is extremely valuable for inactive adults. It permits them to gradually condition their bodies to increased exercise stress without the risk of traumatic injuries which can occur in competitive sports such as basketball, handball, or volleyball. As with any exercise program, however, every individual should take certain precautions and begin slowly.

An excellent feature of jogging is that it can be performed in a wide variety of places. It is best for the beginner not to jog on hard surfaces such as cement or asphalt. If possible, begin running on a track (located at nearly all secondary schools), a grass or dirt path, or on a large smooth grassy area. Varying the place where you jog will add interest to your program. Golf courses, parks, or right-of-ways along parkways can provide good variations in scenery and terrain. During inclement weather jogging can be done at the local YMCA, school or church gymnasium, under protected areas around shopping centers, or even in your own basement. Be sure to give the right-of-way to automobiles, bicycle riders, dogs, and others.

Almost any time of day is acceptable for jogging except for an hour or so after a meal and during the middle of a hot and humid day. It is suggested you set aside a specific time of day for jogging. Early morning before breakfast is often found to be a good time for many people. Such a schedule increases the chances that you will adhere to your jogging program. Also, if you jog with a family member, friend, or co-worker (of similar ability), you will probably maintain a more regular schedule. Jogging with someone else should be for companionship, not for competition.

JOGGING EQUIPMENT

The best guide to use in selecting clothes for jogging is that they be comfortable, reasonably loose, and help keep you cool in the summer and warm in the winter. Women should avoid wearing support garments or clothing that restricts free movement of the arms or legs or impedes the return of blood from the ex-

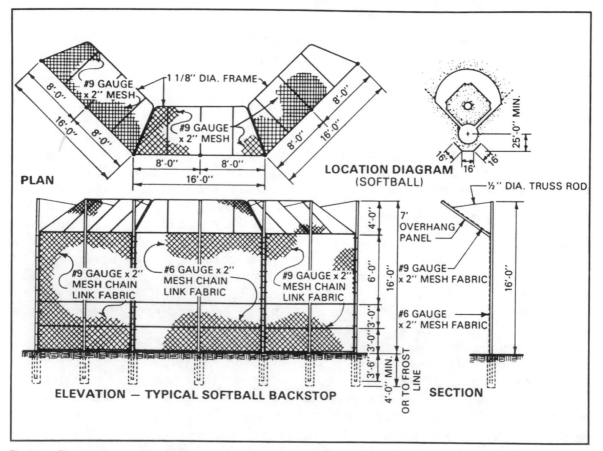

Fig. 9-22. Regulation softball backstop.

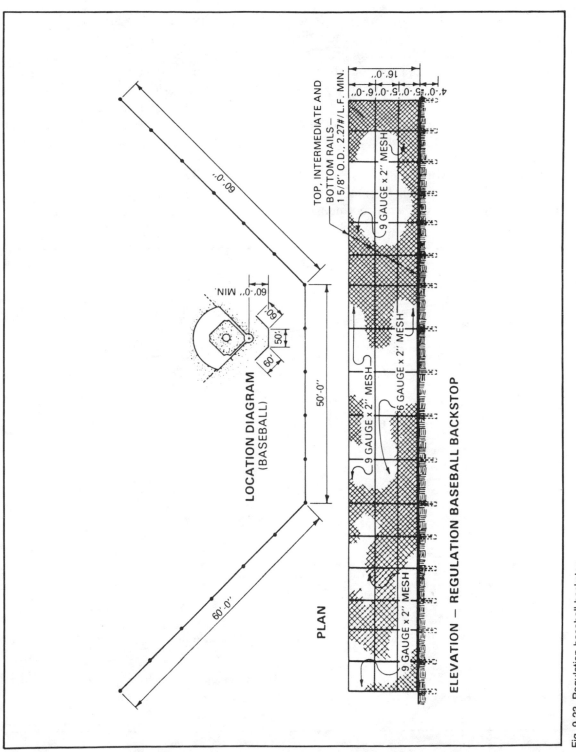

LOCATION DIAGRAM
(BASEBALL)

60'-0" MIN.

PLAN

TOP, INTERMEDIATE AND
BOTTOM RAILS—
1 5/8" O.D., 2.27#/L.F. MIN.

9 GAUGE x 2" MESH

9 GAUGE x 2" MESH

6 GAUGE x 2" MESH

9 GAUGE x 2" MESH

ELEVATION — REGULATION BASEBALL BACKSTOP

Fig. 9-23. Regulation baseball backstop.

tremities. Men do not need to wear athletic supporters while jogging as they frequently cause skin irritations. Workout uniforms or "jogging suits" are not necessary, but they do help motivate some people to keep jogging once they have started.

Don't wear rubberized or plastic clothing while jogging to increase sweating as this will not cause any permanent loss of body weight and can be harmful to your health. Rubberized or plastic clothing can cause body temperature to rise to a dangerous level because it doesn't give sweat a chance to evaporate, which is the principle temperature regulation mechanism for humans during exercise. When sweat cannot evaporate, body temperature increases. This causes more sweating which can lead to excessive dehydration and salt loss resulting in possible heat stroke or heat exhaustion.

Proper shoes are essential for the beginning jogger. A shoe for jogging should not fit too tightly, the soles should be firm, the tops should be pliable, and they should have good arch supports. Shoes especially made for long distance running or walking are highly recommended and are available at most sporting

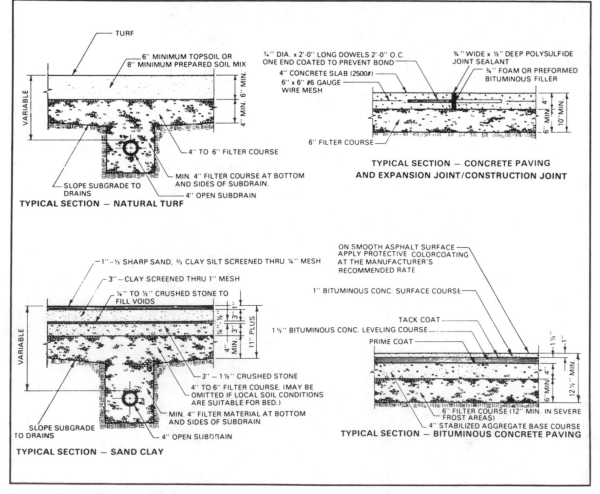

Fig. 9-24. Typical playing surfaces.

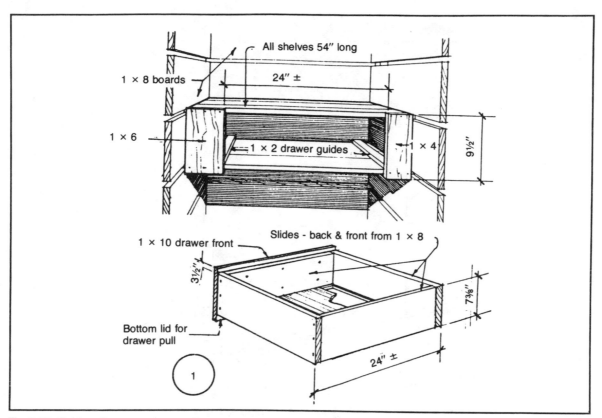

All shelves 54" long

1 × 8 boards

24" ±

1 × 6

1 × 2 drawer guides

1 × 4

9½"

1 × 10 drawer front

Slides - back & front from 1 × 8

3½"

7⅜"

Bottom lid for drawer pull

24" ±

1

Fig. 9-25. Outdoor fitness center stow-it-all storage drawers. (Courtesy Western Wood Products Association)

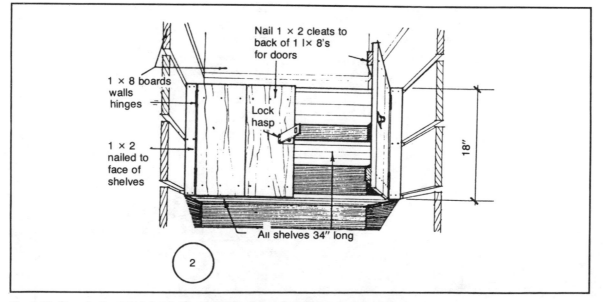

Nail 1 × 2 cleats to back of 1 I× 8's for doors

1 × 8 boards walls hinges

Lock hasp

1 × 2 nailed to face of shelves

18"

All shelves 34" long

2

Fig. 9-26. Stow-it-all cabinet detail. (Courtesy Western Wood Products Association)

191

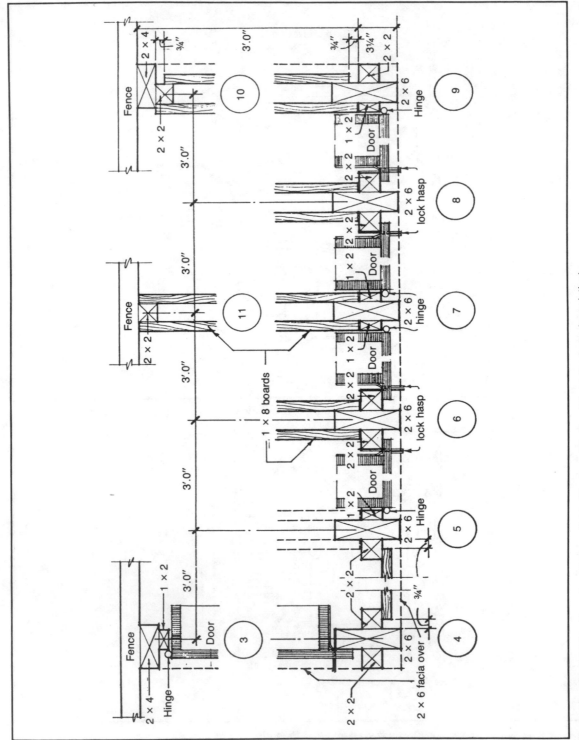

Fig. 9-27. Stow-it-all framing, steps 3 through 11. (Courtesy Western Wood Products Association)

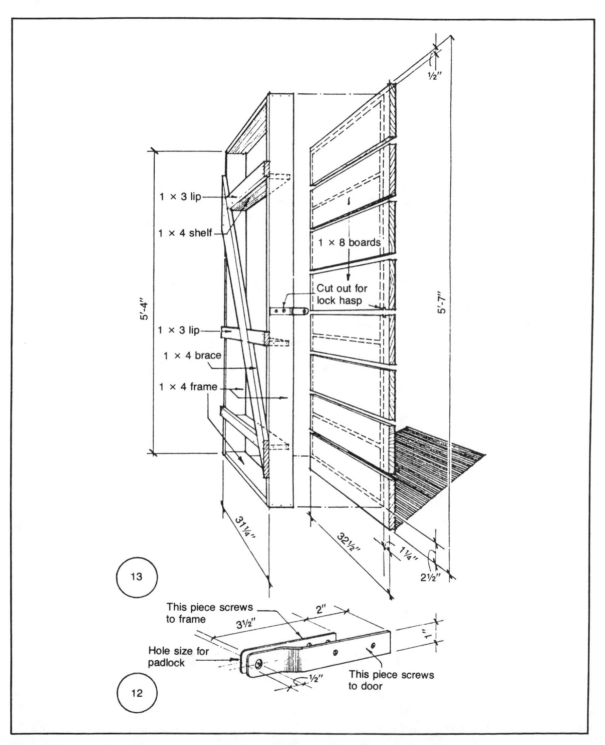

1 × 3 lip

1 × 4 shelf

1 × 8 boards

Cut out for lock hasp

1 × 3 lip

1 × 4 brace

1 × 4 frame

½"

5'-4"

5'-7"

31¼"

32½"

1¼"

2½"

13

This piece screws to frame

2"

3½"

1"

Hole size for padlock

½"

This piece screws to door

12

Fig. 9-28. Stow-it-all framing, steps 12 and 13. (Courtesy Western Wood Products Association)

193

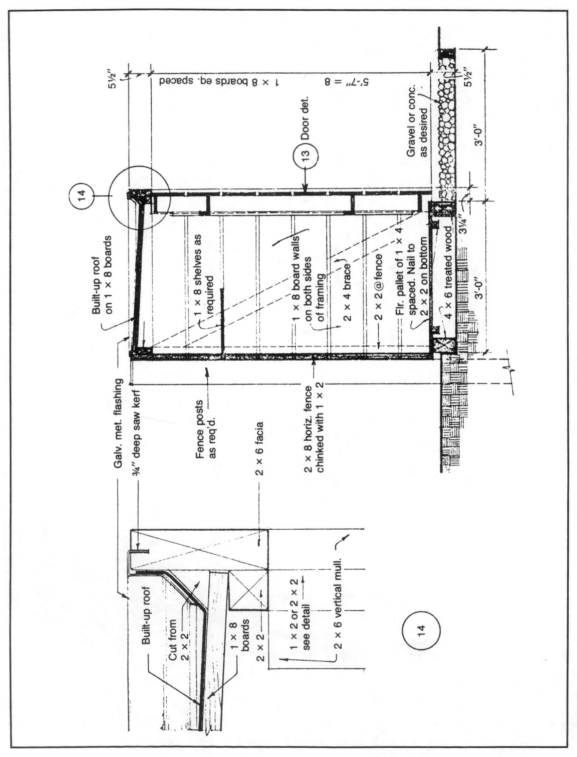

Fig. 9-29. Sectional view of stow-it-all. (Courtesy Western Wood Products Association)

Built-up roof on 1 × 8 boards

14

5½"

1 × 8 boards eq. spaced

5'-7" = 8

13 Door det.

Gravel or conc. as desired

5½"

3'-0"

3¾"

1 × 8 shelves as required

1 × 8 board walls on both sides of framing

2 × 4 brace

2 × 2 @ fence

Flr. pallet of 1 × 4 spaced. Nail to 2 × 2 on bottom

4 × 6 treated wood

3'-0"

Galv. met. flashing

¾" deep saw kerf

Fence posts as req'd.

2 × 6 facia

2 × 8 horiz. fence chinked with 1 × 2

Built-up roof

Cut from 2 × 2

1 × 8 boards

2 × 2

1 × 2 or 2 × 2 see detail

2 × 6 vertical mull.

14

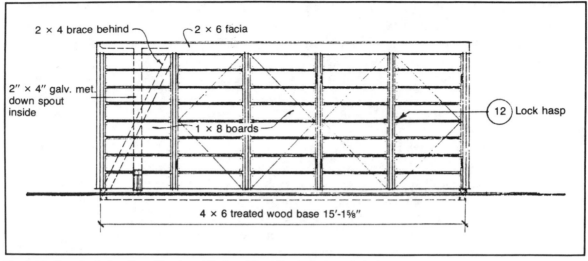

Fig. 9-30. Stow-it-all elevation. (Courtesy Western Wood Products Association)

good stores. Ripple or crepe sole running shoes are excellent, especially if jogging is to be done on hard surfaces such as sidewalks or roads. Inexpensive "gym" or tennis shoes or crosscountry shoes that don't have a well-protected heel or arch support are not recommended for the beginning adult jogger. Remember, good shoes and socks are your best prevention against blisters, sore feet, and aching ankles and knees.

JOGGING TIPS

There is no one correct way to jog. Just as

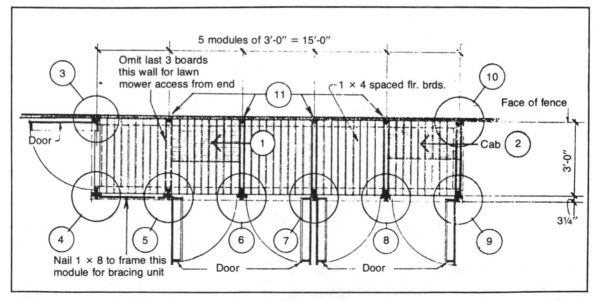

Fig. 9-31. Stow-it-all plan. (Courtesy Western Wood Products Association)

everyone walks in a slightly different way, their manner of jogging will also vary. Here are some general suggestions to follow which will make jogging more enjoyable and will help reduce any muscular or joint soreness that might occur.

First, stand up straight, keep your back as straight as naturally comfortable, keep your head up, and don't look at your feet while jogging. Your arms should be held slightly away from the body and bent at the elbows so that the elbow and hand are approximately the same distance from the ground. Occasional shaking and relaxing the arms and shoulders while running will help reduce the tightness that sometimes develops while jogging or running. Also, periodically taking several deep breaths and blowing them out completely will help you to relax.

A very important part of a successful jogging technique is how your foot hits the ground. There are several acceptable techniques, but the best is to land on the heel of the foot, then rock forward and take off from the ball of the foot on your next step. If you find this procedure uncomfortable or unnatural, try landing on the entire bottom of the foot all at once with most of the weight on the ball of the foot. An attempt should be made to avoid landing just on the ball of the foot because this

Table 9-1. Stow-It-All Materials List for One Module.

MATERIALS LIST FOR SINGLE MODULE			LINEAL FEET
DOOR			
LIP	1 X 3		8
SHELF—SIDES			
& BRACE	1 X 4		30
FRONT	1 X 8	(32½″ LONG X 8 = 21′-8″)	22
WALLS	1 X 8		144
MULLIONS	2 X 6		24
MULLIONS	2 X 2		42
MULLIONS	1 X 2		6
BRACES	2 X 4		18
FLOORING	1 X 4	9 PIECES @ 36″ LONG	27
NAILER	2 X 2		3
BASE	4 X 6	PRESSURE TREATED	12
	OR 2-2 X 6 NAIL-LAMINATED		
ROOF			
SHEATH	1 X 8		15
NAILER	2 X 2		3
NAILER	2 X 4		3
FACIA	2 X 6		14
ADDITIONAL MATERIAL FOR INTERIOR SHELVES AND DRAWERS— SEE MATERIAL LIST FOR ENTIRE UNIT (VERIFY)			
PAIR OF 3½″ BUTT HINGES			
1 LATCH AS PER DETAIL 12			
28 GA. SHEET METAL FLASH AS REQUIRED			
Courtesy Western Wood Products Association			

Table 9-2. Stow-It-All Materials List.

STOW-IT-ALL MATERIALS LIST (WITHOUT FENCE) FOR FIVE UNITS
(ALLOWS FOR BRACES AND VERTICAL SUPPORTS REQUIRED @ BACK WALL TO REPLACE FENCE)

DOORS			LINEAL FEET
SHELF LIP	1 X 3	8 L.F. X 5	40
SHELF & BRACE	1 X 4	30 L.F. X 5	150
FRONT	1 X 8	22 L.F. X 5	110
WALLS	1 X 8		360—*120
	2 X 6		72—36
MULLION	2 X 2		114—36
	1 X 2		30
BRACES	2 X 4		60—30
*PARTITION @ BACK	2 X 4	+ 12 L.F. @ WALL OR FENCE CONDITION	+ 12
ROOF			
SHEATH	1 X 8		72
NAILER	2 X 2		16
NAILER	2 X 4		16
FACIA	2 X 6		39—*16
FLOORING	1 X 4	27 L.F. X 5 = 135 + 2 EXTRA 3′ PIECES	141
NAILER	2 X 2		30
BASE	4 X 6	PRESSURE TREATED	38
INTERIOR STORAGE UNITS			
SHELVES	1 X 8	*4 BOARDS AVERAGE EACH MODULE 36″ LONG	60
DRAWER (EACH)	1 X 8	SIDES 8 L.F., BOTTOM 6 L.F.	14
	1 X 10	DRAWER FRONT	2
	1 X 2	SIDE GLIDES	4
CABINET	1 X 8	FRONT	6
FRONT (EACH)	1 X 2	STYLES	9

*INDICATES MATERIAL NOT REQUIRED WHEN UNIT BACKS UP TO FENCE OR WALL

MISCELLANEOUS HARDWARE
45″ X 1″ X ⅛″ GALVANIZED STEEL CUT AS PER DETAIL 12   5″ X 36′ 28 GA. GALVANIZED FLASHING AS PER DETAIL 14
5 PAIR 3½″ BUTT HINGES—MAIN DOORS   2″ X 4″ X 6′ GALVANIZED METAL DOWN SPOUT AND LEADER
2 PAIR 2″ BUTT HINGES—LOCKED CABINET

Courtesy Western Wood Products Association

will create unnecessary foot and leg soreness. Regardless of what method is used, keep your steps short by letting the foot strike the ground beneath the knee instead of reaching it out in front of you. The slower the rate of running, the shorter your stride length should be.

Remember to breathe deeply while jogging; don't hole your breath. If for some reason, known or unknown, you become unusually tired or uncomfortable while jogging, take it easy and slow down, walk, or stop.

Jogging offers one distinct advantage over many other exercise programs: the whole world is your outdoor fitness center.

FUTURE FITNESS

In the coming years, fitness will be an increasingly important part of our lives as we desire to maintain strong physical health while living in a world that constantly takes physical exertion away. It is very important that we maintain our God-given bodies in good condition with regular exercise, rest, and good foods. Building your own fitness center will help you sustain a regular fitness program that offers both fitness and fun.

Appendices

Appendix A
Fitness Center Sources

Alfra Associates
140 Horton Avenue
Port Chester, NY 10573

Almost Heaven Hot Tubs, Ltd.
Rt. 5 South
Renick, WV 24966

Amerec Corp.
P.O. Box 3825
Bellevue, WA 98009

**American Playground
Development Company**
P.O. Drawer 2599
Anderson, IN 46011

American Plywood Association
Box 11700
Tacoma, WA 98411

AMF American Athletic
200 American Avenue
Jefferson, IA 50129

AMF Inc.
P.O. Box 1126
Wall Street Station
New York, NY 10268

AMF—Whitely Division
29 Essex Street
Maywood, NJ 07607

Anderson-Thompson Leisure Products
1803 S. 124th St.
New Berlin, WI 53151

Caldera Spas
1080 W. Bradley Ave.
El Cajon, CA 92020

California Hottub
60 Third Ave.
New York, NY 10003

Cascade Hot Tubs
P.O. Box 3
Spokane, WA 99210

Warren E. Collins, Inc.
220 Wood Road
Braintree, MA 02184

Diversified Products
309-A Williamson Avenue
Opelika, AL 36801

Dynamics Health Equipment
Manufacturing Co., Inc.
1538 College Avenue
South Houston, TX 77017

Exercycle Corporation
667 Providence Street
Woonsocket, RI 02895

Finlandia Sauna Products
9475 S.W. Oak St.
Portland, OR 97223

Florida Hot Tubs, Inc.
4639 State Road 84
Ft. Lauderdale, FL 33314

Georgia-Pacific Corp.
133 Peachtree Street, N.E.
Atlanta, GA 30303

Great Northern Hot Tubs, Inc.
P.O. Box 273
Osseo, MN 55369

Helo Saunas From Finland
Box 1339
Minnetonka, MN 55343

Hydro Spa Inc.
P.O. Box 377
Piru, CA 93040

ITT Marlow
445 Godwin Ave.
Midland Park, NJ 07432

Jacuzzi Whirlpool Bath, Inc.
298 N. Wiget Lane
Walnut Creek, CA 94596

Jenn Whirlpool Bath
P.O. Box 7671
Boise, ID 83707

MacLevy Products Corporation
43-23 91st Place
Elmhurst, NY 11373

National Equipment
Manufacturing Corp.
12099 44th St. N.
Clearwater, FL 33520

New Life Sauna and Leisure Products
2600 John St., Unit 206
Markham, Ont. Canada

Pearl Baths, Inc.
6801 Shingle Creek Parkway
Minneapolis, MN 55430

Physique Apparatus
P.O. Box 34
Lebanon, NJ 08833

Sequoia Tubs and Spas
4844 E. Speedway
Tucson, AZ 85712

Sunbeam Leisure Products
Howard Bush Drive
Neosho, MO 64850

Sweetwater Manufacturing, Inc.
W220 N1560 Jerico Ct.
Waukesha, WI 53186

Texas Imperial American Inc.
P.O. Box 878
Tyler, TX 75710

Universal Gym Equipment
930 27th Avenue
Cedar Rapids, IA 52803

Vico Products Mfg. Co.
1808 Potero Ave.
S. El Monte, CA 91733

Weider Health and Fitness
21100 Erwin Street
Woodland Hills, CA 91367

Western Wood Products Association
1500 Yeon Building
Portland, OR 97204

York Barbell Company, Inc.
P.O. Box 1707
York, PA 17405

Appendix B
Fitness Organizations and Resources

Aerobic Dancing

Aerobic Dancing, Inc.
18907 Nordhoff St.
Northridge, CA 91328

Bicycling

Bicycle Touring Group of America
21 Grove Place
Rochester, NY 14605

Bikecentennial
P.O. Box 8308
Missoula, MT 59807

League of American Wheelman
P.O. Box 988
Baltimore, MD 21203

United States Cycling Federation
1750 East Boulder
Colorado Springs, CO 80909

Bowling

American Bowling Congress and Women's International Bowling Congress
5301 South 76th Street
Greendale, WI 53129

Hiking/Camping/Backpacking

Forest Service
U.S. Department of Agriculture
Information Office
P.O. Box 2417
Washington, DC 22013

National Campers and
Hikers Association
7172 Transit Road
Buffalo, NY 14221

Sierra Club
530 Bush Street
San Francisco, CA 94108

Running/Jogging
American Running and
Fitness Association
2420 K. Street, NW
Washington, DC 20037

Skating
Roller Skating Rink
Operators Association
7700 A Street
Lincoln, NE 68501

United States Figure
Skating Association
20 First Street
Colorado Springs, CO 80906

Skiing
American Water Ski Association
P.O. Box 191
Winter Haven, FL 33880

Ski Touring Council
c/o Lewis Polak
32 Harmony Road
Spring Valley, NY 10977

United States Ski Association
P.O. Box 100
Park City, UT 84060

Softball
Amateur Softball Association of America
2801 NE 50th Street
Oklahoma City, 73111

Swimming
Council for National
Cooperation in Aquatics
P.O. Box 1574
Manassas, VA 22110

Tennis
United States Tennis Association
Education and Research Center
729 Alexander Road
Princeton, NJ 08540

Volleyball
United States Volleyball Association
1750 East Boulder
Colorado Springs, CO 80909

Walking
Walking Association
4113 Lee Highway
Arlington, VA 22207

General Fitness Organizations
American Alliance for Health, Physical
Education, Recreation and Dance
1900 Association Drive
Reston, VA 22091

American College of Sports Medicine
1440 Monroe Street
Madison, WI 53706

American Volkssport Association
Suite 203
Phoenix Square
1001 Pat Booker Road
Universal City, TX 78148

**President's Council on
Physical Fitness and Sports**
400 Sixth Street SW
Room 3030
Washington, DC 20201

Women's Sports Foundation
195 Moulton Street
San Francisco, CA 94123

**Young Men's
Christian Association (YMCA)**
Check your local telephone directory for the
YMCA nearest you.

**Young Women's Christian
Association (YWCA)**
Check your telephone directory for the YWCA
nearest you.

RESOURCES FOR SPECIAL GROUPS
**American Athletic
Association for the Deaf**
3916 Lantern Drive
Silver Springs, MD 20910

**Blind Outdoor
Leisure Development, Inc.**
533 East Main Street
Aspen, CO 81611

**National Handicapped Sports
and Recreation Association**
Capitol Hill Station
P.O. Box 18664
Denver, CO 80218

**National Wheelchair
Athletic Association**
Nassau Community College
Garden City, NY 11530

**National Wheelchair
Basketball Association**
110 Seaton Building
University of Kentucky
Lexington, KY 40506

Special Olympics
1701 K Street NW, Suite 203
Washington, DC 20006

**United States
Association for Blind Athletes**
55 West California Avenue
Beach Haven Park, NJ 08008

Index

Index

Edited by Steven Bolt

OTHER POPULAR TAB BOOKS OF INTEREST

| TAB | TAB BOOKS Inc.

Blue Ridge Summit, Pa. 17214

Send for FREE TAB Catalog describing over 750 current titles in print.

TUNNELS OF TERROR

Weekly Reader Children's Book Club presents

TUNNELS
OF TERROR

Patricia Edwards Clyne

Illustrated by Frank Aloise

DODD, MEAD & COMPANY
NEW YORK

Library of Congress Cataloging in Publication Data

Clyne, Patricia Edwards.
    Tunnels of terror.

    SUMMARY: While searching for hidden treasure, five young
people find themselves trapped in an underground cave by rising
flood waters.
    [1. Caves—Fiction]   I. Aloise, Frank E., ill.
II. Title.
PZ7.C6277Tu   [Fic]   74–25515
ISBN 0–396–07073–6

Printed in the United States of America

Weekly Reader Children's Book Club Edition

For Frank
who loves Pompey's Cave
best of all

Author's Note

Although this book is a work of fiction, there is an actual Pompey's Cave, and TUNNELS OF TERROR is based, in part, on adventures experienced by my family while exploring this fascinating cave. Special thanks are due Mr. Bob Presbery, who grew up in the area and was kind enough to direct me to Pompey's Cave.

Contents

10

TUNNELS OF TERROR

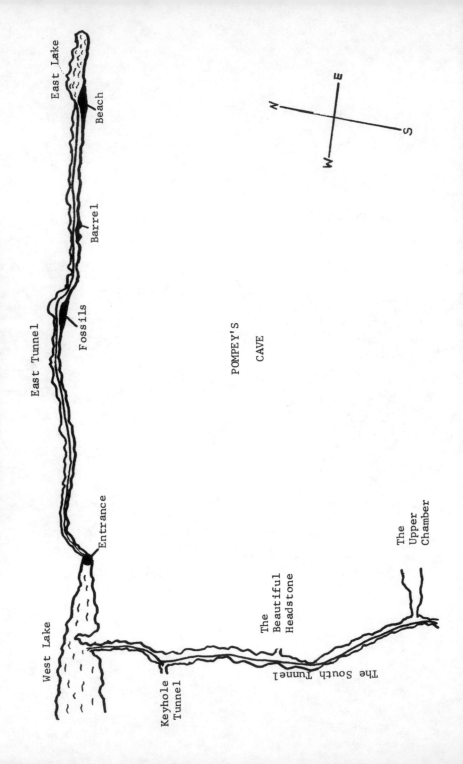

1

Bumblefoot Tags Along

The layered gray clouds appeared cemented to the forested hills—unmoving, unchanging. Below them the lone dirt road ran straight through a gap in the hills, as if anxious to get out of the wilderness area that comprised the northern section of High Falls Park.

Two boys stood in the middle of the road, looking up at the gray shroud above them. Finally, the shorter one asked, "Are you sure it'll be alright?"

Roy Benedict adjusted a loose strap on his backpack before he answered the boy who had arrived only a few minutes ago. "Of course I'm sure Andy," he said. "It's been cloudy like this for the past three days and it hasn't rained yet, has it? Any-

13

way, nobody calls a game just because it *looks* like rain."

"But the radio said . . ."

"A possibility of rain," Roy finished the sentence. "Only a possibility, Andy. But that doesn't bother me. Even if it does rain, we have the ladder to get out before the cave starts to fill up."

Roy's arm suddenly shot out, pointing toward the girl sitting on a rock at the edge of the road. "What does bother me," he went on, "is *her*."

Andy's eyes plummeted to the hard-packed dirt of the road, and his voice held embarrassment as he sought to explain the presence of his ten-year-old sister Sue.

"She blackmailed me, Roy. I had to bring her along."

A whistling breath escaped from Roy's lips. "Blackmailed you? How?"

"Last night Sue found the photocopy you made of that old newspaper article, and she figured out where we were going. She knew Mom and Dad wouldn't be too keen on the idea, so she threatened to tell them if I didn't take her along too."

When Roy turned away from him with an exasperated snort, Andy grabbed his arm.

"Look, Roy, I'm sorry, but I couldn't help it. Anyway, you have some explaining to do yourself.

14

What about you inviting that Edison nut, Bumble-foot, along?"

Roy spun around angrily. "That Edison nut just happens to be the only guy we know who's got a rubber life raft. And it's pretty hard to paddle across an underground lake without one. Furthermore . . ."

A call from down the road cut off his words and both boys smiled when they saw the slim blonde girl approaching them. Then Roy's smile froze when he realized who was with her.

"How come you walked out here with him?" he demanded, gesturing at the boy with a heavy canvas backpack.

"I wanted to show the newest member of the science club where I found the Indian pipe," Alana O'Malley explained. "You know, those plants I brought in for the exhibit on Indian medicines."

"Couldn't you have just told him?" Roy persisted.

The girl grinned up at him. "Why, Roy Benedict, you sound like we were going steady or something."

"It's not my fault that we aren't," Roy joked back, his irritation disintegrated by the glints of laughter in Alana's blue eyes.

Playfully punching the newly arrived boy on the

15

shoulder, Roy said, "Good to have you on the team, Bumblefoot."

"Yeah," Andy put in, "even if we have to listen to stories about Thomas Edison all the way through the cave."

"No Edison today," promised Bumblefoot, whose real name was Chad Evans. "In fact, I've never read anything about Edison even being interested in fossils."

"Fossils!" came a startled shout. "I thought we were going down in Pompey's Cave for lost treasure!"

None of them had noticed that Sue Gregorio, Andy's little sister, had come over to them. But now it was impossible to ignore the excited ten-year-old as she jumped up and down.

"There is a treasure, isn't there, Roy? That article I read on Andy's desk—it mentioned a treasure down there in the cave. We're going to find it, aren't we?"

Chad's face was puzzled as he asked, "What treasure is Sue talking about, Roy? I thought we were going fossil-hunting."

The two other boys exchanged glances, then Roy explained, "Sure, we're going for fossils. The story about a bootlegger using the cave and hiding a treasure down there is probably just an old legend. But there're fossils down there for real!"

16

"Fossils—phooey!" came Sue's declaration of disgust.

But Chad's eyes were gleaming. "A fossil collection would be great for next month's science fair at school, Alana."

"It sure would!" she exclaimed, then eyed Chad quizzically. "But would a lofty ninth grader like you be willing to go partners on such a project with a lowly eighth grader like me?"

Before Chad could answer, Roy groaned loudly, "Science! Science! Is that all you ever think about, Alana?"

"Well, if I'm going to be a scientist someday..."

"I think you'd be a better football player's wife," Roy abruptly stated. Then he turned with a challenging look toward Chad. "Did you bring the raft, Bumblefoot?"

"Right here," Chad assured him, patting the canvas backpack he was carrying.

"In there?" Sue sounded unconvinced.

"It's not inflated, silly," Andy grumbled to his sister. "We'll do that when we get to the underground lake."

"And if we don't break up this huddle, we'll never get there," Roy reminded them as he headed toward the woods at the north side of the road.

There was no actual path, but a so far rainless

17

October had withered the underbrush to make walking easier, and they were soon scrambling down the sides of a dry creekbed.

"Wow!" Alana exclaimed, looking around at the rough-surfaced ledges of sedimentary rock that walled the leaf-covered creekbed.

"If you think this is something, wait till you see the cave," Roy promised her.

The ground was uneven beneath their feet and Roy warned them to step carefully, for the rustling layer of autumn leaves could hide cracks in the limestone that made up the floor of the ancient creekbed.

"What happened to the stream that used to flow through here?" Chad questioned. "The steep sides make it appear that the water must have been too deep to just dry up."

"Your scientific deduction is correct, Mr. Edison," Roy answered. "The article I found said the creek went underground thousands and thousands of years ago. Probably the ground shifted or something, causing cracks in the bed."

"You mean we could fall through a crack where we're walking?" Sue asked, her gray eyes wide.

Roy looked at her quizzically. "Even if I said yes, you'd still come along, wouldn't you?"

"Yep!"

"I figured that," he nodded, then shrugged in

acceptance. "Okay, you're a member of the team now. So I might as well tell you the truth. There are no large cracks that you could fall through, Sue. Just small ones, plus the opening to the cave itself—right over there."

At first none of the others saw it, for it was hidden between two shelves of rock about three feet high. Then Chad spotted the pole sticking up between the rocks, and he hurried over to examine the opening. The others followed, gazing down into the dark narrow hole from which the sound of running water could be heard. It was Sue who spoke first.

"I can see why you didn't tell Mom and Dad the truth, Andy."

"I didn't lie to them!" Andy defended himself. "I told them we were going to a cave in High Falls Park."

"You just didn't mention which one," Sue reminded him. "You knew they'd think you meant that shallow rock shelter south of here."

"How would I know that?" Andy asked, falling into the pattern of bickering that he and Sue had developed almost from the time she had learned how to talk.

" 'Cause they don't even know there's another cave here, that's why!"

"I still didn't . . ." Andy began, but stopped when Roy stepped between them.

"Hold it, you two," Roy ordered. "Just remember, Sue, that what your parents don't know is the very reason why you got to come along with us."

Sue grinned up at him and nodded. She knew better than to bicker with Roy. Anyway, as she had once confided to him, it wasn't much fun to bicker with someone—that is, unless it was with her brother Andy.

Roy couldn't help grinning back at the pint-sized girl who was always there on the sidelines cheering when he and Andy played football for the school team. Then he pointed to the pole sticking out of the hole in the ground. "Come on, team," he urged. "The Pompey's Cave Expedition is now under way!"

2

Into the Depths

"It looks like it goes straight down to China," Sue said excitedly, as she knelt to peer into the hole.

"Only twenty feet on the way to China," Roy laughed.

"That's still pretty far down," Alana commented, peering over Sue's shoulder into the rock-walled shaft. "And that ladder doesn't look any too sturdy."

Roy pretended to be insulted—and perhaps he was a little. "You mean that masterpiece I made last week when I was here? Why, I'll have you know I searched for almost an hour before I found that pole. And it took me at least that long to round up

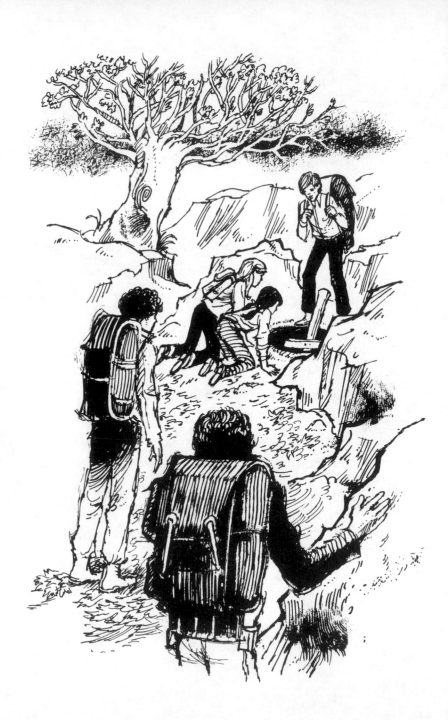

enough wood to nail on as crosspieces. You don't doubt my architectural talent, do you?"

"How could I after that speech?" Alana conceded, but she still gazed dubiously at the ladder.

Taking off his backpack, Roy became serious as he detailed the order of descent. He would go first, followed by Alana, Sue, and Chad. Andy would act as anchor man, handing down the backpacks by means of a six-foot rope. Chad would wait at the halfway point on the ladder, well below the narrow space near the surface. From there he would pass the backpacks on to Roy below.

"Now, remember, only one person on the ladder at a time," Roy cautioned. "And be sure to take off your backpacks before coming down."

"Is the shaft really that narrow?" Chad asked, eyeing the bulky canvas bag which held his inflatable rubber raft.

"Only at the top," Roy answered. "But at that one point I'd never make it if I were wearing my shoulder guards."

Then Roy stepped onto the first crosspiece of the pole that slanted down into the darkness of Pompey's Cave. Before he descended, however, he looked directly at Chad and warned, "Watch your footing on this ladder, Bumblefoot."

Alana could see the muscles tighten in the other boy's jaw and she waited until Roy's head had disappeared below the surface before she asked, "Why does Roy call you Bumblefoot?"

"Because he's always goofing something," Sue answered for him.

"That's not true!" Alana declared. "He's been in the science club since September, and . . ."

"But you're not in their class at junior high," Sue broke in. "So you don't see him as often as Andy and Roy do. Andy's always telling me about the nutty things Bumblefoot does."

Alana gestured for Sue to be quiet, but the young girl wasn't even aware she was embarrassing Chad.

"Ever since he moved here last summer," Sue prattled on, "Bumblefoot's been walking into doors or falling down the stairs. And he darn near blew the opening game with Washington Junior High!"

Alana glanced over at Chad, whose face now looked as if he had a severe sunburn. But he managed a half smile as he tried to explain, "Sometimes I've got my mind on other things."

"Yeah," Andy chimed in, "like Edison." Turning to Alana, he added, "That's all this guy ever thinks of—Thomas Edison and his experiments."

"And what's wrong with . . ." Alana began, but just then Roy's head popped back out of the hole.

"Hey, what are you waiting for? Come on, Bumblefoot, give Alana a hand."

24

Alana glared at Roy. "His name is Chad! Why don't you call him that?"

Roy was defenseless at her sudden attack. "Why, I . . . we've called him that ever since . . . well, he's always fumbling a play of some kind, and . . ."

"Not always!" Alana retorted.

Chad stepped forward, about to say something, but Alana rushed on, "Unless I miss my guess, that's a State Hiking Association patch he's wearing on his jacket—and they only give them out to experienced hikers."

Roy's eyes darted to the red and silver patch on the sleeve of Chad's jacket, then back to Alana. "Oh, that Irish temper!" he groaned, as he drew up his shoulders in mock injury. "Okay, Chad it is." Then he winked. "That is, if I remember." And back down the ladder he went.

It was impossible not to laugh, and even Chad was smiling as Alana began her descent. Part way down the pole, however, she stopped to look at the grooved limestone that was only inches away from her face.

"Did you see these?" she called down to Roy.

"What?" he shouted above the sound of the water, which became louder as Alana descended.

"These grooves in the sides of the shaft—they're as smooth as pebbles on a beach."

"Same reason," was Roy's brief answer, as he

helped her down from the bottom rung of his makeshift ladder.

At first Alana was not aware of the implication of his words, for she was staring in fascination at the small area of the cave illuminated by the weak light filtering down the shaft from the surface.

Then Roy turned on his battery lantern and an eerie feeling of being in another world coupled with the fascination to make her gasp.

They were standing on an island-like conglomeration of rocks in a "room" not more than twenty feet square. To her left, Alana could see that the cavern widened into a larger tunnel with a lake stretching from wall to wall. The waters of this lake were completely still, and aloud she wondered, "Where does the sound of running water come from?"

Roy directed the lantern beam in front of them, where the jumbled rock mass they were standing on came flush with the cave wall. At that point a shallow stream gushed from under the piled-up boulders, its sound magnified by the rock walls. It flowed toward the right, down another tunnel which was narrow and not as high-ceilinged as the one with the lake. However, the stream did not completely fill the floor of that tunnel, and Alana could see it would be easy to walk along the sides.

"What are we going to do first?" she asked.

"Take the raft on the lake over there, or explore the tunnel?"

"That's called the west lake," Roy said. "But it's not the one we're interested in. I didn't go any farther than this when I was here last week. But the writer of the article I read said there's another lake at the end of the east tunnel," and he pointed to the one down which the stream was flowing.

"Hey, are you two kissing down there or something?"

Sue's shout echoed against the limestone walls, causing Roy and Alana to give a startled jump.

"Just a minute, peanut," Roy called, as he turned back to the pole ladder. "Now, come down slowly. Make sure your foot is solidly on the crosspiece before you step on it."

When Alana looked up to watch Sue's descent, she again saw the smooth grooves in the limestone where the rock walls almost met near the opening to the surface.

"What did you mean about those grooves being the same as pebbles on a beach?" she asked Roy.

The dark-haired boy studied her for a second before answering, "In rainy season the whole cave is sometimes filled with water."

"What?" Alana almost shouted.

"Is Roy trying to kiss you again?" came Sue's

27

delighted squeal, as she worked her way slowly down the ladder.

Ignoring the question, Alana turned to Roy, silently demanding an explanation.

"We're mighty lucky," he said quickly, lowering his voice so that Sue could not hear him. "It's not often this part of the country gets such a dry spell. That's why the water's so low in the cave—not a drop of rain has fallen for more than a month. During springtime, I'd imagine this cave is probably full up to those grooves."

"But you said that a bootlegger used to . . ." Alana began.

"What's a bootlegger anyway?" Sue demanded, as she jumped down from the last rung.

"A quarterback who kicks other players in the shins," Roy joked, gently demonstrating what he meant on Sue's blue-jeaned leg.

"Oh, Roy!" Sue complained. "You guys never explain when something sounds really interesting."

"Go sit down on that rock, peanut," Roy ordered, "until you get used to the darkness down here."

As Sue meekly obeyed, her gray eyes wide with wonder at what she saw about her, Roy turned back to Alana. "I guess the bootlegger only used the cave when the water was low."

"Either that or he was an amphibian!" Alana declared.

Roy saw that she was no longer staring uneasily up at the grooved walls. Instead, Alana's eyes kept returning to the tunnel where the stream flowed. The water-carved limestone lay moistly gleaming in the beam of her flashlight, and she didn't even turn around when Chad's voice echoed down the shaft.

"I'm on my way down!"

Twenty feet above the cave floor, Chad and Andy had attached the rope to the first backpack, so it could be lowered past the narrowest part of the shaft.

"Remember to stop halfway down, Bumblefoot. I'll be able to reach you with the rope so that . . ." Andy stopped when he realized Chad wasn't listening to him. "What's wrong?" he asked. "What do you see?"

Lowering his eyes from the leaden sky, Chad murmured, "Oh, nothing. Just thought I felt a drop of rain is all." Then with a quick movement that almost sent one of the backpacks plummeting down the shaft—and which did make Andy groan —Chad swung his foot onto the first crosspiece of the ladder.

The rest of the descent went without a hitch— that is, it did until all the backpacks had been delivered into Roy's waiting arms. Then Chad missed the last rung of the pole ladder and went sprawling on his backside.

Getting up and dusting himself off, he said, "You know, Edison once fell into a culvert when he was racing after a freight train to prevent a wreck."

"What does that have to do with your rump bump?" Andy laughingly demanded, as he reached the floor of the cave.

Chad shrugged. "I dunno. It just popped into my head is all."

"I thought we weren't going to have any Edison this trip," Andy reminded him.

"Well, at least something besides football pops into somebody's head around here!" Alana said, half serious and half joking.

For the second time that day, Roy's dark eyes fastened on Alana, then on Chad, and back again to Alana. All he said was, "It's time we were heading down the east tunnel," but his voice was harsh.

3

Fossil Find

They left some of their things at the base of the pole ladder, taking along only their chisels and hammers, some newspaper, Chad's raft and, of course, their flashlights and Roy's large battery lantern.

Assuming the same order as their descent, they followed Roy along the narrow pebbled ledge between the wall of the east tunnel and the stream. Roy had warned them to keep their heads down, but that was impossible to do when each turn of the tunnel revealed some new and even more fantastically shaped formation. However, when Chad managed to give his head a nasty rap on a protruding rock, each of them was more careful.

"Now I know why spelunkers wear hard hats,"

Chad remarked ruefully, as he rubbed his forehead.

"What's a spelunker?" came Sue's inevitable question.

"An experienced cave explorer," Chad explained. "Obviously something I'm not."

Their laughter echoed hollowly in the tunnel, and Alana suddenly shivered.

"Are we nearly there, Roy?" she asked.

"It should be along here somewhere," Roy grunted, crawling over a slippery slope of rock. "Be careful here—especially you, Bumblefoot."

When there was no answer, Roy turned around. "Bumblefoot?"

"Here. I'm back here," came a voice from behind the bend they had just rounded. "I found some petrified wood embedded in the wall, and I'm going to . . ."

"Come on!" Roy shouted. "That article said there are better things than old wood down here."

"There's treasure!" Sue sang out.

"I was talking about fossils, peanut," Roy corrected.

As Chad and Andy scrambled around the bend, Chad asked, "Are you sure there are fossils, Roy?"

"The guy who wrote the article said the walls of this tunnel contain, and I quote, 'several fossil-bearing layers of sedimentary rock.' "

"Well, I sure would hate to leave that piece of petrified wood behind," Chad told him.

"You can pick it up on our way back," Roy assured him. "But I don't think you'll want to after you've seen what's farther down the tunnel."

"Treasure!" Sue repeated.

"Fossils!" the others chorused—except for Roy. He only smiled at the pony-tailed girl behind him.

"Maybe—just maybe we'll find both," Sue said hopefully, not knowing she was voicing exactly what Roy and Andy had planned from the start.

Before today, however, nothing had been said about the treasure to Chad and Alana. For Roy had told Andy to keep quiet about it because he was afraid Alana might laugh at such an idea. As for Chad, Andy and Roy agreed that the boy they had teased so much might well refuse to accompany them on a treasure hunt based solely on legend. But the definite presence of fossils would guarantee that both Chad and Alana came along—as well as Chad's raft.

Slipping and sliding, they made it over the sloping ledge, then gingerly crossed the now deeper stream on a series of stepping-stones that Roy carefully illuminated for them with his lantern.

"It seems the stream swings left here," Roy explained a few minutes later. "And there's more

33

walking room along this wall of the tunnel. Anyway, the fossils are supposed to be on this side."

Because of the close quarters and the wet rock walls which reflected the rays from the flashlights, they could easily see in their immediate circle. But what lay ahead of Roy's lantern beam was total darkness—just as it was pitch black not many feet behind Andy.

Therefore, they were unaware of the horizontal layer of whitish rock until they were nearly beside it.

"Feast your eyes, Bumblefoot!" Roy cried triumphantly.

A gasp of amazement was his only answer, as the others knelt down to examine the four-inch streak in the darker limestone of the tunnel wall.

It did not need an expert to determine the presence of fossilized shells, for many of them were protruding from their bed of sedimentary rock, as if they could be picked off just like strawberries from a vine. In fact, that was exactly what Sue attempted, only to find that even the barest attachment to the underlying rock made the calcified shells immovable.

"It's like a tiny p-p-putrified beach!" Sue exclaimed.

"Petrified is what you mean," Andy corrected,

34

"but you're sure right. And to think these shells have been here for . . ."

"Since the days of the dinosaurs?" Sue asked excitedly.

"I don't know," Andy replied. "Bumblefoot, what do you think?"

When the other boy didn't answer, Andy turned to see him kneeling on the ledge a few feet away, his flashlight turned on a small book.

Grinning, Chad looked up. "Dinosaurs, did you say? Sue, would you settle for something older?"

Sue giggled. "Oh, Bumblefoot, there's nothing older than a dinosaur!"

"A Murchisonia is," Chad replied, carefully pronouncing the word as he read it from the book. "And that's what I think this is—a type of Paleozoic gastropod 405 million years old!"

The name meant nothing to the other four, but the size of the number did. So chattering excitedly, the young people searched the whitish layer for more fossils. When they had located half a dozen, Roy suggested they begin chipping them out. He and Andy then set to work with the chisels and hammer, while Sue and Alana held the lights.

Unaccustomed to this type of work and unaware at first of the fragility of the ancient shells, Roy accidentally smashed the first fossil.

"I'll take care of the Murchisonia myself," Chad

said. Taking a chisel from Andy, he chipped out a narrow shard of rock about eight inches long, with the tiny fossilized shell in the middle.

Following his lead, Roy chipped out several more fossils, which Sue promptly wrapped in the newspaper they had brought along. It wasn't easy work and Roy's forehead was soon damp with perspiration.

"Let's call time," he said finally. "The few others we can see are too deeply imbedded in the wall. We'd only break them."

Chad nodded. "No need to be greedy. Anyway, I've found a leaf imprint on the other side of this rock shard. So we may have more fossils than we counted on—enough, anyway, to make a fine exhibit at the science fair."

Andy was about to lift the backpack containing the newspaper-wrapped fossils, when Roy gestured for him not to. "We'll pick them up on the way back."

"Back from where?" Chad asked.

"From the underground lake," Roy answered.

"And treasure!" Sue reminded them.

4

The Lake at the
End of the Tunnel

The tunnel widened slightly as they resumed their journey, with the stream running faster and deeper —something Chad found out when he accidentally stepped off the ledge on which they were walking single file.

"Boy, that's cold," he commented. "I can feel it right through my rubber boot."

"If you'd flash your light where you're walking, you wouldn't wind up in the stream," Andy pointed out, with just a touch of sarcasm.

But Chad was again beaming his light on the walls and ceiling. "Judging from those cracks," he murmured, "whenever it rains this place must be like a car wash."

Only Andy, who was right behind him, heard what Chad had to say. "That makes me feel great," he mumbled, "considering what the sky looked like before we came down here." And he shuddered.

As if sensing Andy's reluctance to continue, Roy called back, "We're almost there. I can see that up ahead this ledge widens out and becomes a kind of beach."

"Oh, dear, and I forgot my swimsuit," Alana quipped, and they all laughed.

The joke helped to relieve the tension Andy felt, and he was glad he had gone along when they rounded a water-worn boulder and the lake reflected the rays from their flashlights.

A small beach of sandy silt extended about five feet from the tunnel wall on their side to the stream bordering the other wall. The fast-moving stream emptied into a lake which seemed to fill the rest of the tunnel, yet the mist-laden waters were strangely motionless.

Sue was the one who expressed the feelings of each of them when she announced in a subdued whisper, "It's spooky."

"Of course it is," Roy answered teasingly. "After all, it's the home of Big Pompey."

"Whose home?"

38

Roy laughed. "I'll tell you about him later, peanut. Right now, we've got to inflate the raft." Then he added to Chad, "I hope you remembered to bring along the air pump."

Alana watched knowingly as the sandy-haired boy's left eyebrow raised slightly and his lips compressed to a thin line. But Chad made no remark as he finished unfolding the yellow rubber raft, then reached into the canvas bag for the hand pump.

Taking turns, the three boys soon had the raft inflated, and dragged it into the water. Since it only held two people and there was but a single oar, Roy promptly assumed the role of guide and told Andy to climb in.

"We'll check out what's down there," he said, pointing into the darkness beyond the beam of their lights.

"Be careful, Roy," Alana almost whispered.

The raft crunched against the silty bottom as Chad pushed them off. Then he stood holding the lantern to illuminate as much of the lake as he could.

The light beam extended far enough, he soon discovered, as Roy slowly paddled out over the still water. For the tunnel narrowed, with the ceiling only a few feet above the water along the sides, until it abruptly ended about two hundred feet from the beach.

"This is crazy!" Andy blurted out. "The stream

empties into the lake, yet the water here is perfectly still. Where does the water go?"

Roy's shoulders lifted in a shrug. "I don't know. Maybe underground. But you're wrong about the water being still, Andy. Just watch."

Lifting the oar out of the water, Roy sat motionless. Slowly, the raft swung around in an almost invisible, whirlpool-like current.

"That," Roy added, "gives me the idea that the water probably goes beneath this wall somewhere below the surface. You know, like water going down the drain in a bathtub."

"Is anything wrong?" came Alana's worried voice from the beach.

"We're okay," Roy called, as he dipped the oar back into the water and started paddling.

As soon as they had ground to a halt on the beach and Andy had come ashore, Alana clambered aboard the raft.

"You be careful," Sue cautioned, as Roy began paddling out into the misty lake. "I still think this place looks like something out of a monster movie."

"I told you it's because Big Pompey lives here," Roy answered, deepening his voice in a fairly good imitation of Boris Karloff.

"Big Pompey is a giant snake-lizard," Roy went on. "He lives here in the underground lake guarding the treasure of Bootleg Brody."

40

"Roy, that's just baloney!" Sue accused, but her tone was not as positive as her words.

"You should have read all of that article, Sue," Roy called out. "Some people say Big Pompey is as huge as the Loch Ness monster over in Scotland. But nobody knows for sure, because anyone who's ever seen him has . . ."

"Gotten the hiccups," Alana supplied, in an attempt to end Roy's teasing of Sue.

But Roy went on with his voice eerily coming over the still waters, "That's why it's called the Lost Lake of the Dead."

The maniacal laughter that followed his announcement made Sue's skin crawl. But she didn't let Roy know this. Instead, her voice rang out, "Hey, Roy, I think you've got your dates mixed up. Halloween's not until next week!"

Giving up in defeat, Roy chuckled as he paddled back to the beach and Alana got out. "Your turn next, Sue," he offered.

"No, thanks," she stated.

"You're not afraid of Big Pompey, are you?" Roy teased.

Sue shook her head violently. "Of course not, because there's no such thing! I just don't want a boat ride. I want to find the treasure."

"By the way, you never did tell us much about the supposed treasure," Chad reminded Roy.

41

"There's not much to tell," Roy admitted, "except what's in that old newspaper article." Searching through his pockets, Roy brought out a brownish slip of newsprint he had found in a scrapbook in his grandfather's attic. Then he began to read it:

It was on March 4, 1928, that James Brody was arrested for storing illegal whisky in the depths of Pompey's Cave. While everyone knew Brody had amassed great wealth from his bootlegging operations, none of it has been found. Nor is it likely that any of it will ever be recovered. For three hours after his capture, Brody died from wounds sustained while trying to escape from Federal agents.

"So you think Brody left his money down here?" Chad asked.

"The author mentions the possibility later on in the article, and he says a lot of other people searched for it too," Andy spoke up. "But if the treasure's here, it looks like the only place it could be is down at the bottom of the lake—and I sure don't intend going diving in *that*!"

"Speaking of the lake," Roy said, almost too casually, "If you want to go out in the raft, Bumblefoot, you'll have to do it alone. My arms are tired of paddling."

"Sure, okay," Chad agreed. Then with one foot in the raft, and shoving with the other, he expertly launched the craft and drifted off across the dark waters.

"You did that on purpose, Roy Benedict!" Alana accused. "You thought he wouldn't go out there alone."

When Roy only winked at her with a "Who, me?" look, Alana walked to the edge of the beach, following Chad's progress with the beam of her flashlight. Meanwhile, the boy in the raft had found out it was not easy to paddle at the same time he was trying to light his way across the murky lake.

"Chad, watch your head where the ceiling gets lower," Alana warned. "If you want to put your flashlight in your pocket, I'll go get Roy's lantern and aim it at you. It's stronger than mine."

"Thanks," Chad called. "I'd like to see what's growing under this ledge."

Without a word, Roy handed over his lantern.

As soon as Alana had returned with it, and Sue had added her beam too, Chad pocketed his own flashlight and leaned precariously over the side of the raft.

"Watch out," Alana called, for she could see the doughnut-like edge of the yellow raft crumple under the weight of Chad's upper body.

"It won't capsize that easily," Chad answered,

and leaned even farther out, trying to reach something below the water lapping against the wall on the far side of the tunnel.

Chad had been correct in his estimation. The life raft didn't capsize. But the single oar slipped over the lowered edge of the raft and quickly dropped out of sight beneath the surface of the lake.

"Oh, no!" Alana groaned. "What's he going to do, Roy?"

The dark-haired boy stood beside her, his expression a mixture of amusement and something else which Alana couldn't quite determine.

"Help him, Roy!" Sue cried. "Help him before Big Pompey gets him!"

"I thought you told me there's no such thing," Roy reminded her.

"Don't worry, Sue. I'm okay," Chad's calm voice drifted over the water.

As he said this, the raft was caught up in the invisible currents of the lake. The raft began going slowly round in a circle—a circle that was being drawn toward the end of the tunnel.

"Watch out!" Sue shrieked.

"Be careful of those sharp rocks on your left!" Andy shouted.

"Do something, *please*!" Alana screamed.

But if there was panic on the beach, there was

none in the raft. Looking behind him at the end of the tunnel, then down at the whirlpooling water, Chad calmly lowered his hand into the lake.

Paddling strongly with his cupped right hand, he propelled the raft to the side of the tunnel, then used the uneven walls and low ceiling to push himself the two hundred feet back to the beach.

As the others gathered around him, openly expressing their relief, even Roy could not help voicing a grudging compliment. "You're a cool one, Bumblefoot," he said. "Now do you mind telling us why you were leaning over the edge of the raft in the first place?"

"Just this," Chad said, holding out a dripping, spongy growth with long white "fingers" and dark brown, seaweed-like roots.

"Ugh!" was the general opinion.

"What did you want to grab that for?" Andy asked.

"Well, I'd never seen anything like it before," Chad explained. "And you never can tell when a plant might be valuable. Did you know Edison discovered that synthetic rubber could be made from goldenrod?"

"Here we go again," Andy groaned. "Off the track, as usual."

"I say we get back on the track and head for

where we left our lunch," Roy stated, and began deflating the raft.

Within minutes they were on their way back, the fossil-hunters delighted, the treasure-seekers disappointed.

5

The Mysterious Barrel

"I sure could use some lunch," Andy said, when he took his place as anchor man in the single-file line. "Why didn't we bring the sandwiches with us instead of leaving them by the ladder?"

"Same reason why we left the fossils where we did—less weight to carry," Roy replied over his shoulder. "But let me tell you, my stomach's growling too."

However, lunch was to be delayed still further when they came upon a huge slab of limestone which took up much of the rocky stream bank on their side of the tunnel. Earlier, they had been so intent on reaching the lake, they had failed to see they could get past the rock on the side nearest the tunnel wall. This time Roy noticed it, and gestured for the others to follow.

Actually, it would have been easier to go past the rectangular slab on the stream side. But this other way was different, so they squeezed into the narrow space between the limestone and the wall from which it seemed to have separated in some age long past.

Emerging at the other end of the slab, Sue tripped over a stone, causing her to reach up for a handhold. As her flashlight swung high, it momentarily spotlighted the upper wall and ceiling. But it was long enough for Sue to catch sight of something wedged in between a ledge and one of the many cracks and fissures which scarred the wall of the tunnel. Almost afraid of what it might be, Sue poked Alana before aiming her flashlight beam upward again.

"Why, it's just an old barrel," Sue muttered in disgust, as the others paused to throw their beams on the object.

"But what a size!" Chad exclaimed, climbing up on a rock for a better view. "And is it old—and rotten," he added.

When he had climbed back down, the others noticed the puzzled look on his face. "There's something funny about that barrel," he said slowly.

"How so?" Roy asked.

"Doesn't the size of the barrel kind of make you wonder how it got down here?"

48

Alana was the first to grasp his meaning. "The shaft!" she exclaimed. "The entrance shaft is too narrow for the barrel to go down!"

Chad nodded, admiring the quick mind of the girl he thought was the loveliest in the whole school —in the whole world, for that matter.

"Then how did it get here?" Sue wanted to know.

"Maybe there's another entrance to the cave," Chad speculated.

Roy vigorously shook his head. "No, there isn't. That article gives the whole history of the cave right from its discovery in the 1840's, and the author doesn't mention a thing about a second entrance."

"It's possible that there was another entrance not generally known."

"You mean one that a bootlegger would use?" Andy asked excitedly.

Before Chad could answer, Roy spoke up. "Okay, so it's possible. There's also the likelihood the barrel was built right down here. In any case, I want a closer look at it. Who knows, Bootleg Brody might have hidden his money in it."

The ceiling wasn't too high at this point, and several smaller boulders were piled up along the wall. So Roy easily climbed up to where the barrel was partly wedged in the shallow triangular fault. Then as the others beamed their flashlights up toward him, Roy quickly wiped away the mud still clinging to the ancient oaken staves.

Sue was unable to stand still, and she bounced up and down, with fingers crossed on both hands. "Is the treasure there, Roy? Is it?"

Just as she said this, the barrel came crashing down at their feet. It didn't splinter or break. Instead, the water-rotted staves just seemed to collapse beneath their rusted iron hoops.

It had happened so fast that none of them had time to scream or jump away, and the barrel missed Andy's rubber-booted foot by a scant six inches. The sudden shock silenced all of them, and they just stood there looking at the barrel until Roy scrambled back down.

"That . . . that crazy thing seemed to move by itself," he panted.

"You probably dislodged it when you were wiping off the mud," Chad reasoned.

"No, I wasn't even touching it when it moved," Roy insisted. "It just went by itself!"

"You mean maybe a ghost pushed it?" Sue asked, moving over closer to her brother.

"Impossible!" Chad declared, aware that the others were becoming jittery. "There's no such thing as ghosts."

"How can you be so sure?" Andy demanded. "Just because your Mr. Edison didn't believe . . ."

50

"On the contrary," Chad interrupted. "Edison was very interested in the supernatural. So much so that in his later years he even built a machine to communicate with the dead."

"You're kidding!"

"That's all very interesting," Roy said impatiently. "But why don't we communicate with this barrel?" His tone was bantering and dispelled the eerie feeling that had come over the group. However, Alana noticed that he warily shined his lantern up to the triangular crack where the barrel had been lodged, as if expecting to see some spectral hand.

When none was visible, Roy bent over the dilapidated barrel, easily lifting several of the sodden staves. The pungent smell of rotten wood filled their nostrils as they aimed their lights on the interior of the barrel which Roy had just revealed.

"Nothing!" Alana said, as she expelled the breath she had unconsciously been holding.

"Absolutely nothing except for some glop," Sue muttered in disappointment.

Chad eyed the dejected Roy with surprise. "You didn't really expect to find something in there, did you?"

Roy only shrugged.

"If that guy Brody did leave a fortune in there, it was probably paper currency," Chad went on.

"And unless it was in a waterproof wrapper, it would have deteriorated long ago."

"You mean that glop inside there might have been a fortune once?" Sue wailed.

"Maybe. Then again, maybe not," Roy answered for Chad.

"Well, just standing here isn't helping my empty stomach," the practical Andy told them. "Why don't we go back and eat our sandwiches?"

Alana nodded. "I think all of us could use some food."

"Not me," Sue told them vehemently. "That empty barrel made me lose my appetite."

Surprised at how much his little sister had counted on finding a treasure, Andy tried to tease her out of her glum mood.

"Well, what do you know. We're being favored today with a performance by the divine Miss Sarah Burnliver." And he bowed in front of Sue. "May I have your autograph, Miss Burnliver?"

"I'll autograph your head with a rock if you don't shut up!" Sue retaliated.

"Come on, my gloomy little treasure-hunter," Roy urged, taking her hand. "You'll feel better after we have lunch."

Whatever Sue muttered in reply was lost in the sound of the onrushing stream as they plodded back toward the entrance of the cave.

When they stopped to pick up the fossils they had chipped out earlier, Sue was still forlorn.

"I'll tell you what, Sue," Chad said. "When we finish showing the fossils at the science fair, we'll let you take them to your school as a special project. I'll even help you make a report. How's that?"

The gloom disappeared immediately. "Would you really, Bumblefoot?" Sue asked.

He nodded, then said, "I certainly will help you, but only on one condition."

"What's that?"

"Forget that nickname the football team gave me."

Gray eyes sparkling, Sue solemnly placed her hand in his. "It's a deal, Chad."

6

A Fateful Mistake

"Hey, who put Alana's backpack right on the edge of the lake?" Roy asked in annoyance when they arrived back at the ladder.

"It must have been you, Bumblefoot," Andy accused. "Except for the one we used for the fossils, I never touched the backpacks after I handed them down to you."

"And I handed them to Roy," Chad reminded him.

"Well, I wouldn't have put one so close to the water. Look at it. The bottom's all wet. I just hope the sandwiches are okay."

Alana then untied the strings of her lightweight nylon pack and took out the sandwiches she had made. Fortunately, they were well wrapped in plastic and had remained dry. However, the two boxes of chocolate chip cookies were a soggy mess.

While they were eating, Roy continued to study the backpack. "I still can't understand how it got wet," he mumbled. "Somebody *had* to move it!"

"Maybe there's high and low tide in this cave," Alana joked, never realizing how very close to the truth she was.

"Or maybe Big Pompey came and moved it," Sue said softly. But it was hard to tell whether she was joking or serious.

"You know, I thought I heard something before," Andy said. "A sort of rumbling sound."

"That's only the stream," Roy told him.

"No, it was different than the sound the stream makes. It was . . . oh, I don't know."

Alana got up suddenly, "This conversation makes it mighty easy to start imagining things down here. Even I felt goose bumps when Sue mentioned that snake-lizard. How in the world did that story get started anyway?"

Roy shook his head. "The article only said Big Pompey supposedly guards Brody's treasure. But the legend might even go back to the time when the cave was a station on the Underground Railroad."

"Underground Railroad?" Sue repeated. "You mean a subway like they have in New York?"

56

"No," Roy laughed. "The Underground Railroad wasn't a real railroad."

"Then why'd they call it that?"

Roy proceeded to explain that during the days of slavery, certain people banded together to help slaves escape to Canada, where they would be free.

"The whole operation," he continued, "was called the Underground Railroad—not that it really was underground, but because it had to be kept secret. The escaped slaves would be given shelter and food at various places along the route to Canada. These places were called stations, and Pompey's Cave was one of them."

While Roy spoke, Sue had become very serious, and there was no sauciness in her tone when she asked, "But why was it called Pompey's Cave? I thought Pompey was an old-time city in Italy. We read about it when we were studying volcanoes in science class."

"That was *Pompeii*, not Pompey," Andy corrected, with the exhausted patience big brothers often exhibit.

"And Pompey was the name of the man who discovered the cave way back in the 1840's," Roy went on. "He used it to hide two escaped slaves—a woman and her baby."

"And did they make it all the way to Canada?" Sue asked eagerly.

"The article didn't say whether they made it or not—just that they stayed here for almost a week."

Sue jumped up, pouting. "I don't like stories without a happy ending. In fact, that story doesn't have an ending at all. Maybe the author just made it up."

"It's possible," Roy agreed. "But that's enough history for now. Who wants to go back down the east tunnel with me?"

Andy was yawning—the two hero sandwiches he'd eaten had made him sleepy. "Why do you want to go back down there again?" he asked without much interest.

Roy's brown eyes studied them all for a few minutes before he said, "We looked inside the barrel, but not in the crack where it had been wedged. What if Brody's fortune is up there and the barrel was just used to mark the spot?"

Four pairs of eyes intently met his, and even Andy had stopped yawning.

"I'm game," Chad spoke up. "Quite truthfully, I doubt if there's any treasure there, but at least I can chip out that piece of petrified wood I saw."

The others—now rested and full of food—nodded their agreement, and set about cleaning up the remains of their lunch. While they did so, Roy suggested, "Why don't you take this bag of fossils topside, Andy? We'll be tired enough when we

58

get back and it'll be one less thing to carry up. But be careful of the ladder."

"Might as well take my backpack too," Alana said. "Maybe it'll dry out a little before we head home."

"I still don't understand how it got wet," Roy muttered, but his words went unnoticed in the sudden flurry of activity.

"I'll take my raft up too," Chad was saying. "Have you still got that rope, Andy?"

"Sure, but for what?"

"How do you think we're going to get these packs past the narrow part of the shaft?" Chad asked.

"I hadn't thought of that," Andy admitted.

"If we tie a rope on the pack," Chad explained, "we can keep hold of the other end and just haul it up behind us."

"Kind of like having a dog on a leash."

"Right," Chad nodded. "That way you and the backpack won't be going through the narrow part at the same time."

Andy grinned at Chad. "Now don't tell me Edison did something like that!" But this time his tone wasn't so sarcastic, and Chad grinned back.

When Andy was about five feet up the ladder, the rope he was holding became taut. Then the backpack began moving upward as he climbed.

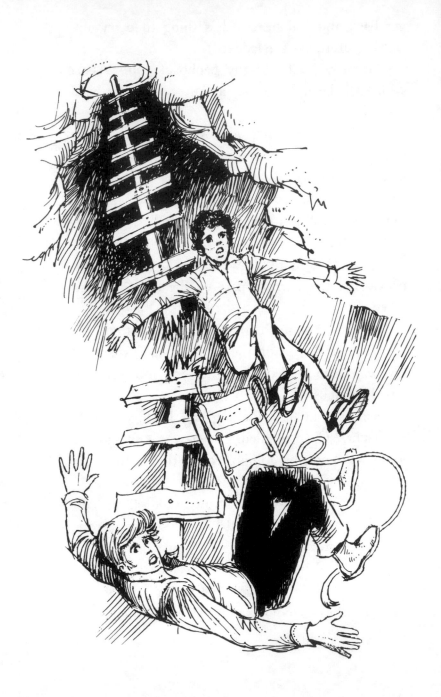

Everything would have gone smoothly if the backpack hadn't swung to the right. But halfway up the ladder it did just that, and as it swung, one of the straps became caught on a crosspiece.

For a few seconds, Andy tugged at the rope. Then realizing what must have occurred, he began backing down the ladder just as Chad started up to unhook the backpack.

At that moment, Roy saw what was happening. He raced over to the foot of the ladder, shouting a warning.

But it was too late. Andy and Chad had already met at the halfway point of the ladder.

There was a fearful splintering sound. Then came an ear-splitting crack as the pole ladder snapped in two, sending boys and backpack thudding onto the rocky floor ten feet below.

7

Trapped!

"My mother often says God protects little children and fools. Boy, she sure is right!"

As he said this, Roy was leaning over Andy, while Alana bathed away the blood on Chad's cheek and hands. Sue held her brother's head in her lap, worriedly staring down at Andy's curly brown hair which now bore a fine film of rock dust.

"Andy's not hurt badly," Roy said gently to Sue. Then his voice became harsh again as he addressed the two boys.

"I can't find any broken bones, Andy. And except for that cut on your cheek," he pointed to Chad, "you don't seem to have hurt your head."

Andy struggled to sit up, pushing away Sue's restraining hand. "Just . . . just the wind knocked out of me," he said hoarsely.

By this time Chad also was sitting up, holding the wet cloth to his scraped cheekbone.

"Of all the fool things you've ever done, Bumblefoot, this takes the cake!" Roy shouted. "I told you the ladder wouldn't support so much weight. But you had to go right on up like super-hero!"

"Roy, stop it!" Alana cried. "Chad went up there without thinking."

"That's pretty obvious!" Roy shot back.

"You might have done the same thing, Roy! Now, why don't you cool down and be thankful that they didn't get badly injured?"

The dark-haired boy glared at her for a moment before stalking over to where the ladder had been. "Keep cool?" he shouted. "Be thankful? Be thankful for what, Alana? That those two fools have trapped us in this cave?"

"Trapped?" It was a mere whisper from the girl's lips, not even audible over the sound of the rushing stream.

"Yes, trapped!" Roy ranted. "That is, unless your boy genius can figure out a way to put the ladder back together!"

Without a word, Chad went over to where the splintered ladder lay like a giant broken bone. A

64

small cold hand pushed into his and he looked down to see the fear-paled face of Sue.

"You can fix it, can't you, Chad?" she asked hopefully.

"I'm going to try my best," he told her grimly. "And so are the others. Don't worry, Sue, we'll get you out of here."

"I know you will, Chad, 'cause you're awful smart. I also know you didn't mean for the ladder to break, so we can't be mad at you. And as soon as he calms down, Roy will know it too."

Meanwhile, Alana had been speaking quietly to Roy and Andy. The two boys then came over to Chad, while Alana took Sue to the far end of the rocky island, saying something about looking for a flashlight battery she had lost.

"What do you think of it?" Roy asked in a calmer tone, as they knelt to examine the broken ends of the ladder.

"We could try splinting it," Chad suggested.

"With what?" Roy asked. "There's no decent wood down here, and we need the crosspieces to climb up on."

"Not really," Chad disagreed. "If we splint it with the crosspieces, then one of us could shinny up the pole and go for help."

"We could use the rope to strengthen the splint,"

Andy spoke up. "And maybe we can salvage some of the nails."

When they examined the crosspieces, they found all but one of them were broken. Still they had to try.

Since they had a hammer with them, it was an easy job to pry off the unbroken crosspiece. The nails were a different matter, however. Most of them had not been driven in straight to start with and were useless when the boys finally managed to extract them. Yet there were a few good ones—and that was better than nothing, they all agreed.

Andy held the splintered ends of the pole together, while Chad kept the crosspiece in place and Roy hammered home the nails. Then Roy wrapped the rope around the pole as tightly as he could.

"Here's hoping," Chad grunted, as he repositioned the pole toward the entrance hole twenty feet above them.

"You better try to shinny up," Roy told him. "You weigh less than Andy or me."

"How about one of the girls?" Chad suggested. "They're even lighter."

Andy shook his head. "My sister may be a tomboy, but I doubt if she could do that. Anyway, she's only ten and that dirt road outside is practically deserted at this time of year. That means she'd have to hike almost a mile to the highway, and possibly another mile and a half to town. I wouldn't want her doing that alone."

"Then let's see if Alana can do it," Roy decided.

The girl was willing enough, but she couldn't master the way Roy showed her to grip the pole with her knees. She slid back down the pole before she had ascended six feet. Alana immediately started up again, but the harder she tried, the less headway she made. Finally she gave up, landing in a frustrated heap on the floor of the cave.

"I guess it's up to you," Roy told Chad. "Good luck."

Using his knees to grip the pole, just as he had learned in gym class, Chad inched up the pole toward the splinted fracture. For one brief moment, he thought he had made it past the danger point. But then he felt the broken ends shift, straining against the rope which was now slipping out of place. Just as the two pieces separated, Chad managed to jump clear, landing on the cave floor a few feet from the fallen ladder.

"Well, so much for that," he told them from behind clenched teeth.

"Are you hurt?" Alana asked, as she ran over to him.

Chad took a moment to smile at her, then returned his gaze to the broken pole. Someway . . .

somewhere . . . somehow there had to be a solution . . .

"Where are the chisels?" he asked suddenly.

"Over there in the backpack. Why?"

Chad was already rummaging through Andy's backpack, pulling out first one chisel, then another, and finally the hammer. "Let's try to chisel out footholds in the wall. Maybe we . . ."

His words trailed off when he saw Roy shaking his head from side to side and silently pointing upward. Following the direction of Roy's finger, Chad's expression became dismal. Then he knelt to replace the tools.

"I hadn't thought about the way the walls arch over toward the narrow part of the shaft," he murmured. "It would be impossible to climb once you got to that point."

"Then what are we going to do?" Alana asked, fear making her voice shrill.

Andy and Chad gestured helplessly, but Roy's eyes lit up when he saw the scarf Alana was wearing. "I've got an idea," he told them. "Give me your scarf, Alana."

The girl quickly complied, as Roy began putting together the broken pieces of the pole.

"If the rope didn't hold the pole together under Chad's weight, do you think the scarf is going to make much difference?" Alana questioned.

"I think we've proved we can't climb the pole," Roy told her. "What I was thinking of was a signal that can be seen from above."

As soon as Roy had securely tied the yellow scarf to the top of the pole which had been splinted again, the three boys maneuvered it into position.

"Now, what do we do?" Sue asked.

"We wait," Roy told her with an optimism he really didn't feel. "As soon as someone sees the scarf, he'll come over to investigate and we'll be rescued."

"How long do you think we'll have to wait?" Sue persisted.

"I don't know for sure," Roy said. "But someone will come soon—very soon."

He could not meet the gaze of the others, which made Chad wonder if Roy was picturing the same thing he was—the dry creekbed many yards away from the deserted dirt road that ran through the wilderness area of High Falls Park.

8

Cloudburst

Only the sound of the rushing stream could be heard as the five dejected young people sat around. Once or twice Andy had raised his head as if listening for something. But he did not say anything to the others.

It was Sue who finally broke the silence. "Gee, wouldn't it be nice if we had a fire," she said hopefully.

"Are you cold, peanut?" Roy asked.

Sue shook her head. "I just thought a fire would be nice and that maybe we could send up smoke signals through the hole."

At first Roy wanted to laugh, but when he realized how serious Sue was, he reached over and patted her arm.

"That's a good idea, Sue. However, we don't have any wood except for our signal pole. And we certainly don't want to take that down. In any event, we don't have anything to chop it up with —no hatchet or ax."

Disappointment washed over Sue's face, causing Alana to suggest, "Why don't you take your flashlight and scout around among the rocks here? There might be some dry driftwood. And you can pick up the broken crosspieces too."

When Sue had scampered away to begin her search among the rocks bordering the west lake, Alana moved over closer to Roy, then gestured for Chad and Andy to follow her.

"How badly off do you think we are?" was her first question.

Roy took a deep breath, then began slowly, "We're in a pretty deserted area, especially now that the summer is over and the campers are all gone. So there's not too much chance of someone passing by to see our flag. As for our parents coming to look for us, I didn't say anything about the cave to my folks. Did any of you mention where we were going?"

Andy was the first to answer. "Just as Sue said, I only told them we were going to the cave in High

72

Falls Park. And of course they'll think I meant that shallow one in the southern section."

"How about you, Alana?" Roy asked.

"My parents were still asleep when I left this morning, so I wrote a note telling them I was going hiking with the gang. But I didn't say where."

"They'll surely be worried when you're not home for dinner, and they'll start looking for you."

"I doubt it."

The bitterness behind those three words shocked the boys. They had never heard Alana say something like that, and they leaned forward expectantly.

"They're so busy with their own lives, they don't pay much attention to my comings and goings," Alana went on. "And since this is the third Saturday of the month, they'll be going to the Archaeology Society meeting tonight, just as they usually do. They probably won't even miss me until they get up tomorrow."

There was nothing any of the boys could say to this, so Roy turned to Chad. "How about you?" he asked.

"I didn't tell my folks where I was going, but I know they'll start worrying if I don't show up for supper."

"Do you think they might call my folks?" Andy asked hopefully.

Chad frowned for a minute. "I doubt it, since they know I usually don't pal around with you. But then again, if I don't come home, they're apt to call everyone they can think of. So at least we know someone will come searching for us." Chad had tried to sound confident, but he knew as well as the others what the chances were of anyone finding the entrance to Pompey's Cave if that person didn't even know the cave existed.

"Hey, what's going on—a powwow without me?" Sue asked, as she dumped a small pile of twigs and broken crosspieces inside the circle the four others had formed.

"I'm afraid it won't make a very big fire," she went on, "but at least we'll have one."

"That's great, Sue," Chad said. "In fact, I think everyone should hunt for scraps of wood. Then we can turn off our flashlights and sit around the fire just like people do when they're camping out."

Sue stood before him with her hands on her hips. "You mean so we can save the batteries in our flashlights, don't you, Chad?"

Made momentarily speechless by Sue's instant grasp of the situation, Chad could only nod, wondering how much she already understood about the danger they were in.

After a futile search for more wood, the five of them sat around the tiny fire, depending only

74

on its flames and the small amount of light filtering down the shaft.

Chad was studying Alana as she gazed into the fire, and he wondered whether her parents were really as unconcerned about her as she said they were. No, he decided, they couldn't be that way —not with anyone as beautiful as Alana.

She's Roy's girl, Chad quickly reminded himself. Then just as quickly he remembered what Alana had said earlier: that she and Roy weren't going steady. Well, when they got out of this predicament . . .

"Say, how about that!"

They all looked up at Andy, who had been watching his sister playing with some of the pebbles that littered the cave floor.

"I was just thinking," Andy went on, "we might be able to build up a pile of rocks high enough to reach the opening to the surface. Then we . . ." His words trailed off when he saw Chad was shaking his head negatively.

"Andy, did you stop to figure out how long or how many rocks it would take to build a twenty-foot pile? That is, *if* we could find enough rocks to build it."

Andy had opened his mouth to protest, but Chad hurried on, "Sure, I know we're in a cave, but just look around you. Most of the rocks are too large and heavy for us to move. It was a good idea, though, Andy."

By now, the small fire had exhausted its sparse fuel and was dying out. Alana and Sue had already turned on their flashlights and Roy was just reaching for his lantern when Chad stopped him.

"I think we'd better conserve the batteries, don't you, Roy? How about just one flashlight on at a time until we get out of here?"

"That reminds me," Andy said, "has anyone got some extra D batteries? Mine have burned out."

"I have two extras," Alana told him. "How many does your flashlight take, Andy?"

"Two's perfect," Andy said thankfully, taking the batteries Alana handed him and inserting them in his flashlight.

"How about your lantern, Roy?" Chad asked.

"I didn't bring along an extra 9-volt battery, but I put a fresh one in this morning."

Glancing at his watch, Chad tried to figure out the amount of battery power they had left. But even though he knew what time they had entered the cave that morning, there were too many variables to make a guess. The only thing they could do was to conserve as much battery power as possible. The others agreed with this idea, and soon Chad's flashlight was the only one to challenge the darkness of Pompey's Cave.

"If it wasn't such a gloomy day, we'd have more light coming down the shaft," Andy began. Then after a brief pause, he asked, "Did you hear that?"

"What?"

"That sound—the one I heard before. I heard it again just now."

"I didn't hear any . . . wait, I do hear something!" Alana said.

They listened intently for a few minutes, but all they could hear was the water in the stream, which sounded even louder in the darkness.

Then all at once the sound came again—a muted rumble barely audible over the noise made by the stream.

"What is it?"

Sue's cry activated Roy, who stood up, flashing his powerful battery lantern over the walls of the cave.

Then they knew.

"Water!" Alana screamed. "There's water dripping down from all the cracks! The cave is filling up with water!"

9

Threat to Survival

For many minutes their frantic shouts drowned out even the rumbling thunder high over their heads. Then an icy terror—even more terrible than their initial panic—froze the cries in their throats. And one by one, they sagged dejectedly to the floor of the cave.

"How long do you think it has been raining?" Roy finally asked Chad.

It was a senseless, unanswerable question and both boys knew it. Still, Chad felt forced to speak. "I don't know, Roy. Maybe from the time I thought I felt that raindrop on my face when we first entered the cave."

"You didn't mention it to me."

"I didn't think anything about it at the time," Chad replied, "because I didn't know then that the cave fills up. Anyway, I think it's been raining for quite a while."

"What makes you say that?" Roy asked.

"That wet backpack—remember? I don't think it was set too close to the edge of the water. I think the lake is rising."

Andy ran his fingers through his brown curls, desperately trying to find another answer. "But if it's raining hard enough for it to come down through the cracks in the cave walls," he said finally, "then why didn't we see it coming down the shaft?"

Chad looked up toward the shaft, where steady trickles of water had now started pathways over the grooved limestone.

"Maybe those ledges on either side of the entrance act as shields if it's a slanting rain. I just don't know," he concluded in defeat.

Alana had managed to control her panic by now, but her voice was strained when she asked, "Wouldn't you think with the ground as dry as it is from the drought that it would soak up all the rain?"

Chad and Roy exchanged glances, remembering what they had been studying in science at the beginning of the term. For a brief moment Chad thought about lying to the frightened girl. But if he did, Alana would find out for herself sooner or later, and then might hate him for not telling her the truth.

Getting up, Chad motioned for Roy to keep Sue occupied while he went with Alana and Andy to where the splinted pole ladder still thrust itself through the entrance hole twenty feet above.

"You asked about the ground soaking up the rain, especially since there's been a dry spell. It's true that usually happens. However, when there has been a drought as severe as the one we've had, the ground hardens like a rock. Then when the rain comes—especially if it's a hard downpour—it just sluices off the ground instead of soaking into it."

Alana's eyes widened in realization. "And what makes it worse," she managed to choke out, "is that this cave lies under an old creekbed that has very little soil. Just rocks—rocks with cracks in them!"

They broke off their conversation as Sue approached them, having tired of Roy's all too obvious attempts to keep her occupied while the others talked.

"What did you decide?" she asked.

"Nothing so far," Andy told his sister. "But we're in no real danger."

The ten-year-old girl eyed him with an expression of scorn. "Andy Gregorio," she said firmly, "you're a liar!" Then she began sobbing.

While Alana tried to comfort Sue, Chad paced the narrow confines of the cave. He was on his third lap past his canvas backpack when he halted abruptly, then dove into the bag for the inflatable raft.

He had already attached the air pump to the valve, when the others noticed what he was doing. Roy was puzzled for a moment, then shouted, "That's a great idea! Why didn't I think of it?"

Seeing the bewildered faces around him, Roy's words tumbled out in a rush. "If the water gets too high in here, we'll just put Alana and Sue in the raft, while the three of us hang onto the sides. As the water rises, we'll float up to the entrance hole. Then we'll be able to climb out."

There were resounding shouts of joy, and Andy began clapping Chad on the back, congratulating him for such a marvelous idea. Then suddenly they realized Chad was unsmilingly shaking his head.

"That wasn't my idea, Roy," he said slowly. "Although we might have to do that as a last resort."

"Last resort? That's our *only* resort!" Roy argued.

82

"No, there's one other possibility," Chad told him. "There's the west lake."

"What about it?"

"We haven't looked over there yet. There might be another opening to the outside."

Roy snorted, "Remember, I told you the article didn't say anything about one."

"And I said that doesn't mean there isn't one," Chad countered. "And I'm going to find out."

With his fists clenched, Roy advanced toward Chad. "No, you're not!" he announced. "You're not taking our only means of survival. Who knows what might happen out there? You could capsize the raft, or run into a sharp rock, or . . ."

"Roy, why don't we sit down and talk this over?" Alana's voice was surprisingly calm. "At least let's hear what Chad has to say."

Reluctantly Roy lowered his fists and motioned toward the spot where the embers of their small fire still glowed.

"Okay, Chad, let's hear it."

With four pairs of eyes intently watching him, Chad groped for the words that would convince them he was right.

"Now, first keep in mind that the cave might not fill up with water this time. But whether it does or it doesn't, I think we'd better try to find another way out. Which brings me to the barrel we found down in the east tunnel. Now, we know it couldn't have come down the shaft here."

Roy was about to say something, but Chad had already anticipated his question.

"I know, we did consider the possibility that the barrel could have been made down here. But the more I thought about it, the more unlikely it seemed. For one thing, barrel hoops were made at a blacksmith's forge. Tremendous heat is needed to make iron workable, and I just can't see anyone—especially a bootlegger—setting up a forge down here."

Chad paused for a moment to see whether he had made his point. He couldn't tell, though, because their faces were as grim as before.

"So figuring that the barrel wasn't made down here, and since we know there are no entrances in the east tunnel, we're left with the west tunnel."

"Not we—*you*!"

When Roy said this, Chad knew the other boy was far from convinced, so he was forced to say the one thing he had hoped to avoid.

"Roy, you think we can stay here, and that by hanging on to the raft as the cave fills with water we'll just rise up to the entrance. But did you ever stop to think how long it might take for the water to rise that high? Maybe hours. Maybe days. Maybe never!"

84

"What . . . what do you mean?" Alana stammered.

"Just because the water *has* risen that high at times doesn't mean it *always* does. What if it stops rising at the twelve-foot level? It'll still be eight feet from the entrance hole. And there'll be twelve feet of water below us. How long do you think you can hang onto the edge of a raft with your body in cold water?"

There was silence in the cave as Chad looked from one to the other, seeing the terror he had induced by his last words.

Finally Roy stood up. "Here, let me help you pump up the raft," he offered. "And you better take my battery lantern with you, Chad."

10

Cold Water, Icy Fear

The four young people stood among the boulders bordering the west lake as they watched Chad paddle off, using his hands in lieu of the oar he had lost earlier.

In an effort to lighten their gloomy mood, Andy called after Chad, "Don't tell me you're setting off without an appropriate Edison quote!"

Chad's chuckle floated back to them across the water. "How's this one?" he asked. " 'The way to find out how to do a thing is to try everything you can think of.' "

"Did Edison really say that?" Alana called, as she beamed her flashlight over the water.

"Yep. I even have that one hanging up over my desk at home."

The word "home" struck them like a physical blow, and there were no more calls between the raft and shore. Only Sue's murmur could be heard as she tightly gripped Andy's hand, "Oh, please . . . please find a way out for us, Chad."

Slowly Chad paddled along the wall of the tunnel, swinging out to avoid the many miniature waterfalls erupting from the cracks, then returning to peer into some dark recess between the huge rock slabs that jutted out into the lake.

Unlike the one they had been in before, the west tunnel had no bends or turns. Therefore, with the water reflection aiding the beams of their flashlights, they could see how the tunnel became progressively wider until it ended about three hundred feet away in a large lagoon-like body of water at least sixty feet wide.

Minute after torturing minute went past as the four on shore watched Chad slowly make his way to the end of the tunnel, circle the lagoon, then start back along the opposite wall of the tunnel.

He was halfway back when they saw him grab hold of a protruding ledge. The beam of the battery lantern danced back and forth across the limestone formations, causing grotesque shadows. Then

88

Chad began back-paddling until part of the raft was hidden behind the ledge.

"What in the world is he doing?" Alana whispered.

No one answered her as they all strained forward to watch. Then suddenly they heard a shout—and Chad's light disappeared!

"Big Pompey's got him!" Sue screamed.

"Baloney!" Roy shouted back, but his voice was hoarse with dread.

Still, he hesitated only a moment before making his decision to plunge into the frigid water of the lake. There was no other choice, though, and he hurriedly slipped off his boots. He was going to swim out past the rock ledge behind which Chad's light had last been seen.

But the slippery footing at the shoreline caused Roy to go crashing into the water on his side. He felt a sickening jolt as his right elbow made contact with a sharp rock. Then his whole arm became numb.

Andy reached him a few seconds later. With his help, the half-stunned Roy rose from the shallow water to make his way back to shore a few feet away.

"Somebody's got to . . . to go find out what happened," Roy said through chattering teeth.

At that moment Chad's voice echoed through the

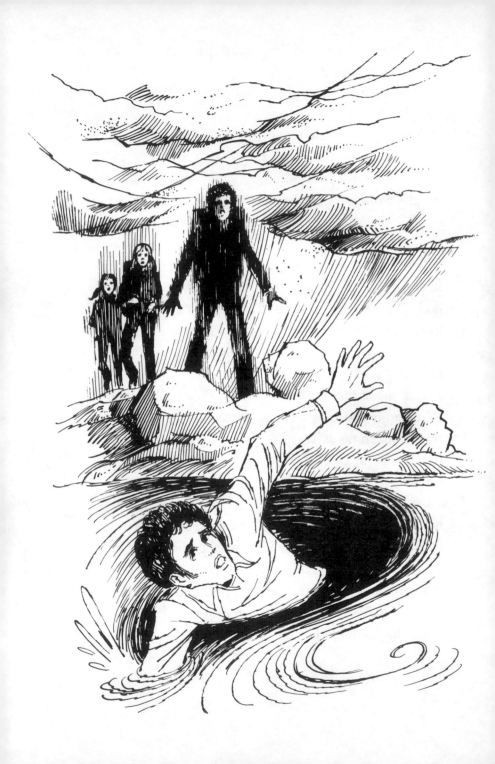

west tunnel. Then the beam of the battery lantern appeared from behind the projecting rock, and Chad quickly paddled the raft along the tunnel wall to where they were gathered.

"I found it!" he was shouting. "I found another tunnel branching off from this one. And it's an *upward-sloping* tunnel, too!"

As soon as he had beached the raft and stepped ashore, Chad was besieged with questions. But by now Chad had spotted the drenched Roy and his jubilant expression turned into one of concern.

"What happened to you, Roy?"

Before the shivering boy could answer, Sue shrilled, "He thought you were in trouble, Chad. So he tried to save you. Only he slipped on the rocks and hurt himself."

"Some rescuer I am," Roy muttered, rubbing his arm.

"A pretty brave one, I'd say," Chad maintained. "Now let's take a look at your arm."

Luckily, there did not seem to be any broken bones. However, as the numbness wore off, Roy's elbow began to throb painfully.

"Try not to use it," Chad advised, as he went rummaging in a side pocket of his backpack. Taking out a heavy fisherman's sweater, he offered it to Roy, saying, "You'd better get off that wet shirt and jacket before you catch pneumonia."

"Now who's rescuing who?"

"Turnabout is fair play," Chad answered. "I only wish I had some dry pants to give you."

As soon as Roy had changed into the warm sweater and had put his boots back on, Chad told them, "I don't know where that other tunnel leads, but I know it's higher than where we are now. What do you think?"

"I think that anyplace would be better than this," Alana promptly voiced her opinion.

"And how!" Sue seconded.

Andy nodded vigorously. "This place is filling up like a bathtub."

All of them shivered when he said this, but Chad still waited until Roy spoke. "I guess it's our only choice," the dark-haired boy finally said.

"Okay, then it's decided," Chad stated. Pointing to the side of the tunnel where the wall met the rising water of the lake, he went on, "There's a narrow, sloping rock shelf just below the surface of the water. I spotted it on my way back. Instead of taking you one by one in the raft to the other tunnel, we'd save time if we waded over there."

"How deep is it?" Andy asked, thinking of his sister.

"I tested it with my hand on the way back. The water was just over my wrist, so it shouldn't be any more than six or seven inches deep."

Sue was already at the edge of the water. "I'm

glad I've got my waterproof boots on," she said. "Now who goes first?"

Sue's decision went for all of them, they agreed. So as soon as Chad had deflated the raft and stowed it in his backpack, they set out across the slippery rock shelf along the tunnel wall.

"Watch your head, and don't try to rush it," Chad warned, as his own foot slid dangerously close to the edge of the shelf.

It was only about 150 feet to the opening of the tunnel Chad had discovered. But they were constantly kept off balance by the silt-slick shelf which sloped sharply down into the lake. In addition, there were places where the limestone wall jutted out and they had to squeeze past these, clinging to the wet rock which offered no secure handholds.

"We'll have to climb over this one," Chad told them when they reached an outcropping that pushed out into the lake about ten feet. "The tunnel is right behind it."

Chad climbed over first, but even with his help the others had difficulty scaling the smooth wet rock.

"Boy, I'm glad that's over!" Alana panted, when the five of them finally stood at the mouth of the new tunnel.

"Me too!" Sue echoed breathlessly.

Chad made no reply. Somehow he knew their ordeal had just begun.

11

Tunnels of Terror

They had paused to rest only a few minutes before entering the tunnel which, in its inky blackness, seemed like some monstrous mouth ready to swallow them up.

Once inside, however, Andy remarked that it was not much different than the east tunnel, except it was wider and the floor seemed to be on an upgrade.

"There's one other difference," Chad said, as he beamed his flashlight on the foaming stream that ran down the side of the tunnel toward the west lake. "Do you see it?"

Roy was the only one who nodded. "The stream here flows into the lake. So if we go up the tunnel, we'll be heading away from where the water collects."

"That's what I figured," Chad said, then turned to the others. "The ceiling of the tunnel is high enough that we won't be banging our heads, so I think we ought to start conserving our battery power again."

Sue stood there with a forlorn expression. "I haven't got any left to conserve," she said, pointing to the darkened head of her flashlight. "It went dead a few minutes ago."

An unwelcome but equally uncontrollable feeling of dread gripped them. *One flashlight dead— how long would the others last?*

"Let's get going," Chad urged, aware of the fear they all felt because it clawed at him too. "We'll just have Roy's light in front and Andy's in back."

It was a relief to start off again, for it was impossible to concentrate solely on their predicament when they had to watch every step they took on the rock-strewn floor of the tunnel.

Because of the width of the tunnel and the fact that the stream did not run down the exact center of it, but more to one side, it would have been easy to walk two abreast. However, they had unconsciously resumed their single-file line, only this time Chad was behind Roy, followed by Alana, Sue, and Andy.

"I figure this tunnel runs south," Roy was saying, just as Chad pulled him to the left. "Hey, what's . . ."

His words stopped abruptly when he saw Chad's finger on his lips. Then Chad whispered, "Watch out for the water coming down."

Guiding Roy's hand holding the lantern, Chad beamed it up to the ceiling. Roy gasped.

Directly above the path of the stream on their right, the ceiling was fractured by jagged, narrow cracks that resembled lightning bolts. Only instead of electricity, water was pelting down. Occasionally an arm of one of these cracks extended over their path, causing a curtain of dripping water to form.

Yet it was not the water alone that made Roy gasp. From either side of the tunnel, the limestone overhead leaned toward the main jagged crack running along the center of the ceiling. It was as if some giant hand was pushing downward on the ancient rock, and the ceiling might fall at any minute.

Chad's hand gripped Roy's, forcing him to lower the lantern. "Just don't let *them* see it," he whispered hoarsely.

But the others were not looking overhead when Roy and Chad turned around. They were staring across the stream at the tunnel wall on the other side. There in the cone-shaped beam of Andy's flashlight loomed still another tunnel leading off from the one they were in.

"What do you think?" Andy asked.

Chad was already splashing across the shallow but fast-moving stream. The top of the other tunnel's keyhole-like opening only came up to his chest, and he had to bend down to inspect the narrow corridor which sloped upward. The thick mud covering its floor, plus the smoothly grooved limestone of its walls, convinced Chad that it was a water course from above. In fact, a small rivulet was already cutting a channel through the mud, then splashing across the pebbles at the opening to join the stream a few feet away.

"What did you find?" Alana called.

"It's like a drainage pipe—and just about as narrow as one," Chad called back. "But I think it's worth exploring a bit. Maybe it leads to the surface where there's a hole large enough for us to crawl through."

Roy was just about to start across the stream to join him when Chad held up his hand. "No sense in all of us getting muddy," he reasoned. "You stay where you are and I'll give it a quick look-see." Then with a wave of his hand, he crawled into the mud-carpeted tunnel.

"Andy, you be careful!"

At Sue's shout, Chad turned his head to find Andy crawling along behind him.

"Just in case you need help," Andy said simply.

However, it was Andy who soon needed help.

They had crawled on their hands and knees at least ten yards up the narrow tunnel when something crashed into Chad's nose. Then a sudden gush of water from above knocked the flashlight from his hand.

Sputtering and choking, unable to turn around or even to move his head out of the spurting water, Chad groped blindly for his flashlight. Raising his other arm to ward off the water, he managed to choke out, "Back up, Andy! Hurry!"

Panicked by the sudden darkness and the urgency in Chad's voice, Andy tried to turn around, only to have his foot become wedged between two shards of rock half buried in the mud.

"I'm stuck, Chad!" he gasped. "My foot! It's caught in some rocks!"

Unable to help the boy behind him and equally unable to get his head out of the gush of water from above, Chad fought hysteria as he shouted half-choking directions to Andy.

"Don't . . . don't try to jerk it . . . out! Try and . . ." His words were lost in wracking coughs.

Ducking his head between his shoulders, Chad

managed to get some relief from the pounding water.

"Point your . . . your toe to the ground," he sputtered. "Then try lifting it out. Don't . . . don't force it!"

Behind him, Andy felt the fear beginning to weaken his legs and he fought against reaching back to wrench at his trapped foot.

"Slowly!" came Chad's garbled voice. "Try it slowly!"

"I can't!" Andy shouted. "It's stuck!"

By this time both boys could feel the water rising up past their knees and wrists. Small twigs snagged at their clothes, and some leaves were plastered against the top of Chad's bowed head.

All of a sudden, the gushing water eased up for a moment, giving Chad time to get some air into his tortured lungs. Just before the water returned to full force, he managed to shout, "If your foot got in between those rocks, then it can come out the same way! Keep trying, Andy! Keep trying!"

Then he began choking again as the water surged over him. There was no way to breathe . . . no way to get out of the relentless downpour . . . no way . . .

Chad was only vaguely aware of the tug on his ankle. His mind was fuzzy and it was hard to concentrate on the words he heard Andy shouting. Then he felt another tug, and he automatically backed up.

"Come on, Chad!" Andy's voice was clearer now. "I got my foot free. You can back up now. We'll be out in a minute."

Only ten yards, but it was like ten miles in the black, narrow confines of the tunnel. The water swirled around their thighs as they crawled backward—one knee behind—then the other knee—push with your hands—back—back—slowly—too slowly!

Chad could feel someone's hands on his shoulders. Looking up, he realized they were out of the keyhole tunnel, crouched on the narrow shelf between it and the stream.

"You okay, Chad?" Andy asked, his worried face a sickly color in the light coming from the other side of the stream.

Chad tried to nod, but was seized by a series of rasping coughs which left his nose and throat feeling like sandpaper.

By that time, Roy had sensed something was wrong and came splashing across the stream to meet them. Andy motioned that he could limp back unaided. So Roy took Chad's arm, helping the still coughing boy to the other side of the tunnel where Sue and Alana waited.

A few minutes passed while Andy related what had happened in the tunnel. But it took longer than that before Chad was able to answer Andy's question as to why the water had suddenly gushed out at them.

Touching the sore spot on the bridge of his nose, Chad finally replied, "A piece of a branch hit me. I caught sight of it just before it struck. It must have been washed down from outside. I guess it got caught crosswise in the place the water was coming through, kind of like a plug. Then when the water in back of it finally swung it around, it shot through the opening."

"That's why the water slowed down the second time too, I guess," Andy said. "Something else plugged up the opening for a while."

"Probably," Chad agreed. "Anyway, we know we can't get out that way." Then he frowned.

"What is it?" Alana asked.

"I just remembered I lost my flashlight in there," Chad said, annoyed with himself. "Boy, I'm a Bumblefoot for sure!"

"Not you—*me*!" Andy corrected. "I'm the one who got his foot caught."

Chad forced himself to smile back, appreciating Andy's gesture of friendship. But his mind was drumming out a distress signal which could not be ignored: *Two flashlights gone—how long will the others last?*

12

A Beautiful Headstone

There was no longer any need to try and keep the others from seeing the water spurting from the cracks in the ceiling. It was only too obvious, Chad realized, as they stared in helpless anxiety at the stream now raging down the incline of the tunnel.

They had paused on the damp rocks opposite the keyhole tunnel in order to give Chad and Andy time to catch their breath. But the drenched boys soon found their teeth chattering uncontrollably, and Chad stood up to shoulder his backpack again. Exercise would help warm them up, and the sooner the better.

"Wait," Roy said. "We can take turns wearing the sweater you gave me."

Alana and Sue looked down at their own heavy sweat shirts, with Sue voicing what both of them were thinking. "How about my sweat shirt?" she asked.

Andy grinned in spite of his chattering teeth. "Not likely, peanut," he said, unconsciously picking up Roy's nickname for his sister. "But thanks anyway."

Alana was already in the process of pulling hers over her head, but Roy stopped her with a gentle hand on her shoulder. "We're football players, remember?"

Chad said, "Give it to Andy first," when Roy took off the sweater and put back on his own soaked shirt and jacket. "Then we better take a look at that ankle he hurt."

However, when Andy groaned as he touched his throbbing ankle, Chad shook his head doubtfully. "We better not take off your boot, Andy. If your ankle is swelling, we might not get the boot back on."

"But if his ankle hurts . . ." Alana began.

"Chad's right," Roy broke in, unaware that for the first time he was using the other boy's real name. "The boot will keep the ankle from ballooning up. We can always cut the boot off when we get outside."

"*If* we get outside," came Sue's doleful voice.

104

The four words pressed down on them like a heavy blanket, smothering any spark of optimism they might have had. Alana slowly slumped back down on the rock where she had been sitting, staring with fear-filled eyes at the stream boiling past them on its way down the tunnel.

"You know," Sue said, speaking more to herself than to the others, "Mom is making hamburgers tonight. I saw it on her shopping list. If I had gone to the supermarket with her this morning, instead of . . ."

Her words trailed off to be swallowed in the noise of the stream, but all of them knew what Sue meant. If they had only done something else today instead of going to Pompey's Cave . . .

"You might still be home in time for those hamburgers."

Chad's voice startled them all, and they turned to stare at him in dull-eyed disbelief.

"Why not?" he challenged. "That is, if we get a move on."

"What time is it, anyway?" Sue asked.

Chad automatically raised his arm, then lowered it without looking at the watch on his wrist. "It got wet in the tunnel, so I don't know the time," he told Sue, hoping he sounded convincing.

Sue was about to ask somebody else, when Roy spoke up. "It's time to get going," he stated, backing up Chad. "Alana, you be our anchor man with the flashlight. Andy, you lean on me—you know, like the time you helped me off the field when the Washington team almost clobbered us. We weren't beaten then either, were we?"

Forcing a grin, Andy put his arm around Roy's shoulder and said through teeth that still chattered, "No, we weren't beaten."

"And we aren't now," Chad echoed, as he picked up Andy's backpack as well as his own.

Andy gestured toward the canvas pack. "Oh, just leave it, Chad. It . . . it doesn't matter now."

For a moment Chad considered the possibility, but the defeated tone in Andy's voice made him decide against it, and he slung the straps over one arm. "You a millionaire or something, Andy?" he chided. "Anyway, carrying this extra weight will work up a sweat—and I sure wouldn't mind sweating some right now!"

The wet pebbles on the floor of the tunnel crunched and skittered beneath their feet, causing them to lurch from side to side as they struggled along. It was no longer possible to avoid the countless showers of water that sprayed down from the walls and the ceiling—nor did they attempt to avoid them. It was hard enough just forcing their tired legs up the sloping tunnel.

Roy and Andy were right behind Chad when they heard the scrambling sound of slipping stones, then a high-pitched "Ow!" as a heavy thud told them one of the girls had fallen.

For a second there was only darkness in back of him as Chad turned around. Then the beam of the battery lantern picked out Alana sprawled among the rocks.

"She's hurt! She's hurt!" Sue cried out, kneeling next to the motionless girl.

But by that time Chad had reached her. Alana was sitting up, her chin wet with blood.

"No, I'm all right," she insisted, brushing away Chad's arm. "It's just a scrape. But the flashlight— oh, Chad, the flashlight!"

Wordlessly, Chad examined the smashed head of the flashlight. He was about to toss it away when Roy's voice stopped him.

"Take out the batteries first," he advised. "We'll have to use Andy's flashlight now, and those batteries will help if Andy's give out."

Chad nodded and went over to Andy, who reached for his back pocket. A puzzled look came on Andy's face, but quickly turned to one of desperation as he frantically searched his other pockets. Then with a groan, he told them, "It's gone! My flashlight's gone!"

"How could you lose it? Where? When?"

Roy's machine-gun questions only made Andy more confused. "I . . . I just don't know."

Meanwhile, Chad had discovered that part of

Andy's back pocket had torn away from the underlying jean material. "It must have happened when we got caught in the keyhole tunnel," he reasoned. "Any other time, Andy would have felt his pocket rip."

"Maybe we could go back and find it," Sue ventured.

"With the way the water was gushing out of the keyhole tunnel, Andy's flashlight might be at the bottom of the west lake by now," Roy muttered.

"Well, after being in the water, it wouldn't have been any good even if we found it," Andy said.

Roy spun around, his dark eyes blazing. "You don't know what you're talking about! A flashlight isn't a candle! And a little bit of water won't put it out!" Then he turned to Chad. "Isn't that right?"

Chad stood there with a grim expression. Roy was right, of course. The dunking in cold water might have reduced its power, but the flashlight would have been operable at least for a while longer. However, there was no sense in adding to Andy's misery, so Chad remained silent.

Alana put one hand on Roy's arm and the other on Andy's shivering shoulder. "What's done is done," she said quietly. "So let's forget it. After all, we might have lost more than just two flashlights in that tunnel."

The unmistakable meaning of her words immediately cooled Roy's anger, and he gripped Andy's shoulder by way of apology.

Still, it was impossible not to be depressed over their loss, and for long minutes they stood there in the weakening light of the battery lantern. The only sound was the noisy rush of the stream on their right. Their only thought: *All the flashlights gone— how long will the battery lantern last?*

Then suddenly Sue shouted excitedly, "But I've still got my flashlight, and all it needs is batteries!"

"You gorgeous peanut!" Roy laughed. "We'd forgotten about that. Chad, load it up with Alana's batteries and let's get going!"

Their spirits revived by the addition of one of the lights they thought they had lost, they once more set out along the tunnel.

There was still a perceptible upward slope, which they could feel in the tired muscles of their thighs, even if they were unable to see it. However, the tunnel appeared to be narrowing and the stream was closer as it raged past them in the opposite direction.

"Hey, what's this?"

The beam of Chad's lantern swept the rock wall to their left, then flashed up.

"It's a passage alright!" Roy shouted.

"And it leads upward!" Alana cried, as she added

the beam of the flashlight to that of the battery lantern.

Together they stepped into the narrow cleft in the wall. A few feet inside, the passageway ended in a steep limestone slope. The two light beams joined, then gradually climbed the wet limestone, only to illuminate a crack a scant four inches wide high above their heads.

Sue had not followed the twin beams all the way up to the slitted rock which terminated their hope of escape. Instead, she was staring at the towering slab of dark limestone, which bore a mantel of lacy white flowstone laid down over the years by the countless drops of mineral-bearing water that had filtered from the rock above.

"Oh, look," she breathed, still unaware of the disappointment the others felt. "It's so beautiful."

"Yea," Roy rasped, without thinking. "A beautiful headstone for a watery grave!"

13

A Message from the Past

Their failure in the keyhole tunnel had in no way prepared them for the despondency that now gripped them. It was impossible to even hope, after the disappointment of what Roy had called their "beautiful headstone."

They were colder now, hungrier, and more tired —especially Sue, who stumbled along behind Chad, her icy fingers firmly clasped in his own chill hand. Behind them Andy limped, supported by the nearly breathless Roy, whose husky body was beginning to tremble from the burden of his friend's weight.

Although their pace had slowed considerably, Alana was finding it harder and harder to keep up with the others. She began to lag behind, first a few feet, and later several yards. Then for one panic-stricken moment she could not see the pale gleam of the battery lantern up ahead, when Chad rounded a slight bend in the tunnel.

"Chad!"

The sound—more of a shriek than a call—echoed against the wet limestone walls. And though it took less than a minute for him to reach her, Alana was shaking by the time she felt his strong hands grip her shoulders.

"I . . . I'm sorry," she managed. "I just can't keep up. Got . . . to rest . . . please."

Fearing they would give up once they stopped, yet knowing all of them were unable to continue without some rest, Chad agreed. The fuzzy tentacles of exhaustion were beginning to strangle his own will to survive.

"Well, at least we're still going uphill," he said after a few minutes.

He was sitting next to Roy on a small shelf near the wall of the tunnel, while the other three had chosen seats a few feet away, but still within the dimming yellow circle cast by the battery lantern.

Roy heaved a long sigh, then looked closely at Chad. "I figure," he said slowly, "that even with a gradual upgrade, we've climbed more than twenty or thirty feet—a lot higher than the opening back where we first entered the cave."

Chad nodded, waiting for Roy's next words.

"I'm thinking about the lay of the land when we were walking along the dry creekbed—about the hill on the side. This tunnel runs south, right?"

"As near as I can figure." Chad's voice was low.

"So that puts us right inside that hill," Roy stated. "We could go on climbing forever!"

"What?"

They had been so intent on their conversation, they hadn't seen Alana come up to them. But now her chalk-white face was only inches away from Roy's. Her wide blue eyes seemed to be pleading with him to deny what she had just heard.

It was Chad, however, who answered her. "Look," he said miserably, his eyes downcast, "I could be wrong. There may not be an opening at the end of this tunnel. I just don't know!"

Gesturing toward the stream which raced even more furiously along the side of the tunnel, he went on, as if to himself, "All I know is that we're heading away from where the water is going. Can't you think of what it's like back there by the ladder?"

Alana's sharp intake of breath revealed that she, too, remembered the water-polished grooves in the shaft where they had entered Pompey's Cave.

"What I'm thinking of," Roy said quietly, "is what if there's no opening at the end of this tunnel? What then?"

Chad gestured vaguely. "Then . . . then we . . ."

"We're trapped!" Alana's whisper hissed through the chill air, the two words biting at them like a snake, spreading the paralyzing venom of terror.

Physically fighting the idea, Chad shook his head violently. Then leaning toward the other two, his eyes as intense as his voice, he said, "Don't you remember the barrel? It had to come from another opening somewhere!"

"Now, you . . ." Roy began, but Chad cut him off.

"I still don't buy that idea about the barrel being made down here. That's just not logical!"

"Is any of this . . . logical?" Alana sighed hopelessly, but Chad ignored her.

"Just think," he insisted. "At a time when the water was high in the cave—like now, or even higher —the barrel could have floated down this very tunnel, into the west tunnel and the lake, past the place where the ladder is, then down the stream in the east tunnel to where we found it."

But the other two weren't really listening to him.

"We've got to try!" Chad urged.

Alana turned away from him to stare again at the dripping walls. "But is it any use, Chad? We've tried and tried and . . ."

"And we've got to keep on trying!" he desperately tried to convince her. He paused a moment,

114

concentrating on something in the back of his mind. Then he rushed on with the only other argument he could think of.

"Do you know Edison tested fifteen thousand different plants before he discovered he could make synthetic rubber from goldenrod? And it took fifty thousand experiments before he perfected a way to improve the storage battery. That's trying!"

A faint smile touched the tired girl's lips, and she began nodding slowly, just as Sue came over to them.

"Are we almost there?" she asked. "I'm awful hungry for those hamburgers."

"Yes, Sue," Chad answered, as he wearily got up from the rock. "You sit here and rest a little longer. I'm just going to scout around."

Before he did so, however, Chad helped Andy over to sit with the others. The injured boy's gray eyes were red-rimmed and he didn't even question where Chad was going.

It was as if he had seen all this rock before, Chad thought hazily, as he forced his eyes to search over the dark and dripping walls. The shadows looked like passageways until you aimed your flashlight straight at them—but they were just shadows.

The limestone assumed strange forms in the roving light, and it didn't take much imagination to see a witch's hat in that protrusion there across the stream, or an Indian's grim profile in the rock right ahead of him, or even an arrow pointing . . .

Chad spun around, almost unbalancing himself on the slippery pebbles beneath his boots. An arrow? The flashlight beam raced back to where he had seen it. There? No, there! It did seem like an arrow—an arrow pointing upward . . .

But Alana, who had been watching him, was the first to stumble over to the limestone slab that formed a corner of one of the innumerable shallow recesses in the tunnel wall. Chad was right behind her, and together they bent to rub their fingers over the long depression in the rock.

"Is it . . . do you think it's real?" she asked breathlessly.

Chad touched it again. "It doesn't look like that was gouged out naturally. It's more like chisel marks."

Alana's blue eyes brightened with a sudden spark of hope. "A chisel? You mean that someone . . . someone scratched that in the rock?"

Chad did not answer immediately, as he traced the line upward to where it ended in what looked like an upside-down "V."

"That *is* an arrow!" he shouted. "And it's pointing to something!"

Rising from his knees, he swung the lantern upward into the shadows of the protruding rocks high

116

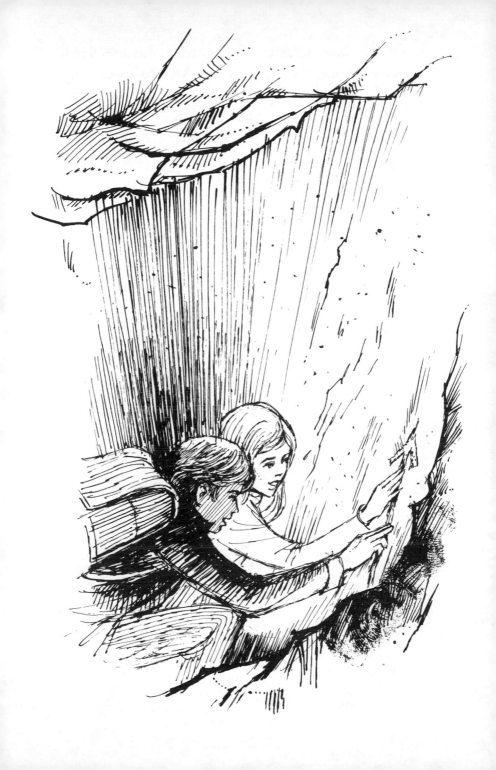

above them. Crevice after crevice was examined. One by one, the shadows gave way to reveal only more limestone. Then one shadow did not yield to the probing ray of the lantern.

"It's another passage! An upper chamber to the tunnel!"

14

Barrier Against Hope

Their excited shouts brought the others scrambling over the rocks to stare up at the gaping hole high above them.

It was Sue, the shortest of them all, who was the first to realize the difficulty involved. Craning her neck back to better judge the distance, she said, "It looks great, but how are we going to get up there?"

Her question was like jerking a TV plug from its socket. The excited voices ceased abruptly, leaving the enthusiasm to fade from their faces more slowly.

Sue was right, of course. At least thirteen feet of water-polished limestone towered above them, "with not a handhold or foothold in sight," Andy observed gloomily.

"You know much about rock climbing?" Roy questioned, eyeing the hiking patch on Chad's jacket.

Chad shook his head. "I was going to take a course in rappelling and prusiking next summer."

"Repelling who?" Sue asked.

"Going up and down rocks with a rope," Roy explained, too preoccupied with the problem to smile at her word mix-up.

"That's right!" Chad exclaimed. "We've got that length of rope," and he was suddenly very glad that he had continued to carry the heavy backpacks.

"Yea, but one of us still has to get up there to attach it," Andy reminded him. "And the rope's only six feet long."

"I know, I know," Roy told him impatiently, then began studying Andy and Chad. "Let's see—you're the lightest of the three of us, Chad," he recalled. "So you'll have to go on top. Think you can climb on my shoulders?"

Chad understood immediately. "I can try."

"Okay," Roy nodded. "Andy, you be the stepladder."

"What are you doing?" Alana asked, but it was soon evident.

The husky dark-haired boy stood with his back to the wall leading to the upper chamber, while Andy bent down on his hands and knees in front of Roy.

120

Chad quickly stepped on the kneeling boy's back, then with a boost from Roy's cupped hands, providing a second foothold, he managed to climb onto Roy's shoulders.

For a second Chad swayed uncertainly. Then he managed to steady himself as he reached for the lower lip of the hole in the wall above him.

Sweat streamed down Roy's face, and the tendons in his neck stood out taut against his shirt collar as he strained to uphold Chad's 135 pounds.

Tautly, Alana and Sue watched Chad's long fingers clawing toward the opening only inches away. Then an explosive breath whooshed through the tense air, and he called down, "No use . . . I can't reach it."

Slowly, Roy let his knees sag, sliding his back down the damp limestone, until Chad could safely jump off his shoulders. Then Roy slumped down to a sitting position, his body trembling from the exertion. "I'm taller," he panted, "but I'm too heavy for either of you."

"Maybe I could sit on Chad's shoulders," Sue offered.

A smile brushed across Roy's lips. "No, peanut," he replied. "You'd only crack your shell."

"Crack!" Chad shouted. "That's it! There are cracks in the rock. We can use the chisels!"

Roy looked up with a frown. "You mean chisel out footholds?" The others followed his eyes as he looked over at the stream which was now beginning to spread across the floor of the tunnel. There was no need for him to add that they did not have time.

"No," Chad told him. "What I was thinking of was hammering the chisels into the cracks. Then we can use the chisels like steps."

Roy nodded in agreement, but Andy reminded them, "We've only got three chisels."

Chad, however, had already thought of that. "You can pull out the lowest one and hand it up to me when I'm standing on the one above it."

The backpacks were quickly searched and the first chisel tapped part way into a crack about three feet high on the wall. Roy then boosted Chad up to stand with one foot on the protruding piece of steel as he searched for another split in the rock. Finally he found one nearly three feet farther up, and slightly to the left. After hammering in the second chisel, he spotted a third crack just above the height of his head and quickly pounded the last chisel into place.

When it seemed secure enough, Chad held on to the topmost chisel and pulled himself up to stand on the middle one. There he waited until Roy was able to free the first chisel and toss it up to him.

It was all going so well that Alana had turned her attention to Sue, helping the younger girl stuff the cuffs of her jeans back into her boot tops. Then suddenly Chad's frustrated cry caused her to look up in alarm.

"I can't . . . I can't find another crack to place the chisel!"

The third chisel was only three feet above the second one, but without a handhold, Chad could not climb onto it. The remaining chisel would have to be placed somewhere near the topmost one—but *where?*

"Forget the chisel if there's no crack for it," Roy urged. "The chisel you're standing on is about six feet up the wall. You should be able to reach up nearly two feet past the top of your head. The edge of the hole is only about that far away. See if you can grab onto the edge. Then you can pull yourself up."

After securing the remaining chisel and the hammer in his belt, Chad began.

Chilled, bruised fingers, the nails ragged from clawing over rock, were extended to their fullest— up, up—only inches more. The edge was there, just above his groping hand. Then his fingers felt it, the tips curling over the rocky lip of the upper chamber.

If he could only pull up—hoist his body the rest of the way. Not far now. Just a little bit more . . .

But it was impossible. He simply did not have enough of a handhold.

Feeling his foot slipping on the chisel, Chad leaned against the dripping limestone. Slowly he allowed his foot to slide forward until the narrow steel bar was secure against the heel at the arch of his boot, much like a stirrup.

The disappointment of defeat made a grim mask of his face when Chad jumped down to the rocky floor where the others stood in solemn silence.

Roy waited only long enough to grip Chad's shoulder in a gesture of sympathetic camaraderie. Then he took the tools from Chad, stuffed the rope in his back pocket, and quickly tapped the remaining chisel in the original hole about three feet above the tunnel floor.

When his full weight touched it, the chisel shifted downward slightly in the crack. Roy's hand automatically shot up to the topmost chisel, which he grabbed tightly in the event the first chisel didn't hold. But it did, and he brought his other foot up to the second chisel, testing it before he lifted his body the rest of the way.

Being taller than Chad, Roy could easily grasp the edge of the upper chamber. But did he have the strength to haul himself up—especially now, with a sore elbow and after the many exhausting hours of slogging through Pompey's Cave?

Breathing deeply several times, the dark-haired boy clenched and unclenched his fists as he sought to limber up the already tired muscles of his arms and shoulders.

"I've got to do it," he murmured. "There's no other way!"

With one last deep breath, he reached over his head.

Down below, the other four watched anxiously. The shirt Roy had put back on was still wet, and clung to the bulging muscles of his shoulders and arms.

Slowly—agonizingly, he pulled himself up, as the toes of his boots vainly sought purchase in the smoothly rounded limestone.

The blood pounded in his temples and there was a painful burning just under his Adam's apple.

All his strength was in his next upward lunge, which placed most of his weight on his right arm. Needles of pain stitched through his rock-bruised right elbow, but he did not falter.

For just a fraction of a second after his lunge, his left arm was lifted above the edge. It was now or never!

A strangled groan erupted from Roy's throat as his left elbow came down hard on the unyielding rocks. But it was over the edge!

Hour-long seconds trudged by as he hung there, one elbow on the floor of the upper chamber, his almost-numb right wrist pushing—pushing.

Then his full weight shifted to the left elbow. His right leg swung up—not far enough. A second swing—higher this time. His knee was over the rim!

He hunched there for a moment. Then his right hand clawed at the floor of the upper chamber, found a solid hold—and he dragged the rest of his body over the edge.

He was inside the upper chamber!

15

The Upper Chamber

Roy had taken the remaining flashlight with him, so that the others had only the yellowing beam of the battery lantern as they waited. Chad kept the lantern trained on the opening above them, hoping Roy would reappear before the others became conscious of the cold water which was beginning to fill the tunnel from wall to wall.

Finally, Roy's matted dark curls could be seen at the edge of the upper chamber. Then his pale face appeared. "Had to . . . to take a minute to catch my breath," he explained, still panting from the exertion of the climb.

"You were great, Roy—just great!" Alana called up to him.

Roy grinned briefly at the compliment, then became serious. "And you're going to have to be great, too, when you see what's up here."

"Why? What is it?"

"Spiders," Roy told her bluntly.

"Ugh!" was Alana's immediate reaction, quickly seconded by Sue.

Chad responded differently. "If there are spiders up there, that must mean there's a passage to the outside!" His statement, however, was based more on hope than on any specific knowledge of Arachnoidology.

"Then I'll gladly join the spiders!" Alana assured them enthusiastically. "How do I get up there, Roy?"

Roy thought for a minute, then answered, "Chad better come first. I'm still pretty winded, and he can help haul you up. Andy, you still our anchor man?"

"Right, Roy," the other boy called. "I may have a bum ankle, but it's not as bad as it was. I can manage."

Cheered by the renewed vigor of the group, Roy leaned over the edge to help Chad, who had already climbed up to the second chisel. Alana wanted to go up the same way, but Roy insisted that once she had gained the second chisel she at least secure the looped rope around her waist in case she slipped.

Aided by Andy, Sue made it to the second chisel,

128

where she caught the loop of rope Chad swung down to her. Once the loop tightened under her arms, Chad hauled her up bodily, amid Sue's loud complaints that she felt like a cargo of bananas. Then Andy followed.

"Have you looked around at all?" he asked the others when he reached the upper chamber.

Roy shook his head. "Only at the spiders."

When Alana shuddered, he pointed the beam of the flashlight toward a recess in the wall near the opening. "At least they aren't black widows. They're brownish, and they seem to be congregated mostly over there."

The flashlight beam revealed a rotting pile of wood.

"Hey, that's not just old branches!" Chad exclaimed. "Look at those pieces. I'll bet anything that was once a ladder."

Alana and Sue hung back, but the three boys moved over to examine the wood. On closer inspection, it did look as if it might have been a ladder at one time, but was now the home of the fuzzy brown spiders Roy had told them about.

"They probably eat the insects in the wood," Chad speculated.

"Or things like *that*!" Andy was pointing at something lying between the wood and the tunnel wall.

Chad knelt down to find the mottled bones of a

small skeleton. "Must have been a dog or maybe even a fox," he murmured. "Probably fell in here and couldn't climb back out. See here?"

Roy moved closer and nodded as the flashlight beam revealed the broken foreleg of the skeleton.

"So there has got to be an opening to the surface from this chamber!" Chad exclaimed triumphantly.

"Maybe so," Roy said quietly, "but will the opening that the animal came through be large enough for humans?"

Chad and Andy looked at him with stricken expressions.

"We've got to face facts, fellas," Roy went on softly, so the two girls could not hear. "It seems to be pretty dry up here, so I think we're fairly safe from the rising water. But if there's no passage from this chamber large enough for us, then . . ."

He left the sentence unfinished, but Chad and Andy were well aware of the rest. If there was no outer passage from the chamber, then they were, indeed, hopelessly trapped. For once the water rose in the tunnel below them, it might be days—maybe weeks—before it went down again.

Their earlier cheerfulness had been replaced by grim determination when they returned to the two girls, and Chad found it difficult to take the ten-minute rest Roy had suggested before they searched the chamber.

130

Alana had agreed to sit down only as long as she was within the light cast by the lantern, "So I can see if there are any spiders nearby," she explained.

Knowing that soon they might have even less light, Chad sought a way to get her mind off the chamber's tiny inhabitants.

"If that *was* a ladder," he began, "I wonder who put it there."

Roy apparently sensed what Chad was doing, for he took up the idea, saying, "Well, we have three candidates from the past: the man who discovered the cave, the escaped slave that hid out here, or Bootleg Brody."

"You think any of them left any food around here?" Sue asked.

"None we'd be able to eat, peanut."

"Well, I sure am hungry. I'll bet Mom is wondering where we are, too."

"I guess she is," Andy agreed.

"You think she and Dad will come looking for us, Andy?" Sue persisted.

"Probably."

"And your folks'll be worried if you're not home soon, Alana."

"I don't think so," the older girl answered, before turning away. Then despite the lack of illumination, she suddenly got up and went over to the edge of the chamber, looking down into the darkness of the tunnel. The sound of the rushing water from below effectively muffled the sobs she could no longer control.

Chad had followed her. Without saying a word, he put his arm around Alana until her shoulders stopped shaking and she was breathing more normally.

"What . . . what you said earlier about your parents," Chad began. "About them not caring—you really feel that way, don't you?"

He could feel her head nod against his shoulder.

"I . . . I wasn't interested in the fossils just for the science fair," Alana said slowly. "I was hoping we'd find some unusual ones that would really impress my parents."

Then remembering that Chad had moved to High Falls only a few months ago, Alana explained, "My father was a field archaeologist. You know, someone who goes to faraway places. My mother used to go with him—that is, until I was born. Then because of me, he took a job teaching at the state college here. But now that I'm older and they can send me away to camp in the summer, they go on short digs by themselves."

"Didn't you ever ask to go with them?" Chad wanted to know.

"They wouldn't want me along!" Alana asserted

132

hotly. "You see, I complicate their life—I don't really have a place in it."

Chad was quiet for several minutes. Then he said, "I guess a lot of kids feel that way about their parents. And some of them may be right. But a lot of them are wrong—just like I was."

"You mean you thought your parents didn't care about you?" Alana asked.

"Well, actually I felt they were disappointed in me, especially after that football game with Washington Junior High, when everybody started calling me Bumblefoot. But it was my father who pointed out that I only have those accidents when I've got my mind on something other than what I'm doing—preoccupied, he called it. Then he told me he was happy with me just as I was, bruises and all."

When Alana didn't answer, Chad went on, "I guess what I'm really trying to say is that if my folks and I hadn't talked together about it, I might have gone right on believing they didn't think very much of me."

"Well, my parents aren't . . ."

Alana was interrupted by Sue calling, "Hey, Roy, you better watch out! Chad's stealing your girl!"

"That Sue!" Alana groaned. "Even when she's trapped in a cave, she . . ."

Suddenly brought back to their present danger, Alana sobbed, "Oh, Chad, I'm scared!"

"So am I," he admitted. Then his voice strengthened. "But that's not going to keep me from trying to find a way out of here. Come on, Alana, let's start searching."

When Chad and Alana rejoined the others, they split up into two groups. Roy took Alana with him, while Chad, Andy, and Sue went down the other side of the chamber to search the spider-filled darkness.

Unlike the tunnels below, the walls of this chamber were made up of massive slabs and columns of rough limestone, with huge boulders piled up as if some giant hand had tossed them there.

The ceiling, when they shined their lights up there, was a jumble of shadowed furrows and knobs, with occasional darker rocks—some studded with shining mica "spangles"—compressed against the predominant limestone.

Time after time, they thought they had found something, only to be brought up short by a barrier of rock. Sue was obviously on the point of exhaustion, and when she complained about climbing up a series of steplike boulders, Andy readily agreed to sit with her while Chad went on.

"But I don't want to stay here in the dark!" Sue protested.

134

Her voice had carried over to Alana and Roy.

"We'll stay with them so they'll have light," Roy offered. "Go on up, Chad."

Within seconds, Chad had disappeared behind a column of limestone, climbing the boulders that leaned against the tall pillar. The lantern beam wavered from one shadowed crevice to another until Chad hit upon what at first looked like a lighter-colored slab of rock high above him.

Strangely enough, this gray patch reflected none of the light from the lantern, and he climbed up several more feet until he could make out what it was. Then when he did, the chamber echoed with his excited shouts, "The sky! It's the sky! We've found the way outside!"

16

Up from the Depths

It was almost as if they had not heard Chad's triumphant shouts. For too many hours they had concentrated on fighting against a growing belief that they would never escape from Pompey's Cave. And now that the impossibility had become a possibility, they were momentarily incapable of accepting it.

Because they had tried to shield her, Sue had been least touched by the hours of peril. However, even she remained speechless until Chad had scrambled back down the steplike boulders. Then the reaction came.

"Whoopee! Me first!"

The little girl's enthusiastic cry activated the

others, and the chamber echoed with the ear-splitting cacophony of five people all shouting and laughing at the same time.

But their jubilation was not so great that they wanted to spend a minute longer than necessary in Pompey's Cave. And by the time Chad had shouldered the backpacks again, Sue had taken his hand, while Roy lent a supporting arm to the still limping Andy.

It was a relatively easy climb over the piled-up boulders—a fact which made Chad worry when, halfway up, he glanced behind him to see Alana still at the base of the boulders.

"You okay?" he called down to where the yellow circle of the other flashlight bobbed over the rocks.

"Be right there," came her cheerful voice. "Just wanted to see something."

Chad was about to ask her what, but at that moment Sue's delighted cry filled the air.

"We're out! We're really outside!"

The hole through which they climbed was wide enough for both Roy and Andy to emerge side by side. Yet not three feet in front of them a chest-high boulder blocked the way, causing them to separate until they had rounded this last barrier.

They were standing on the crest of a hill. Above them—seemingly so close they could touch them—

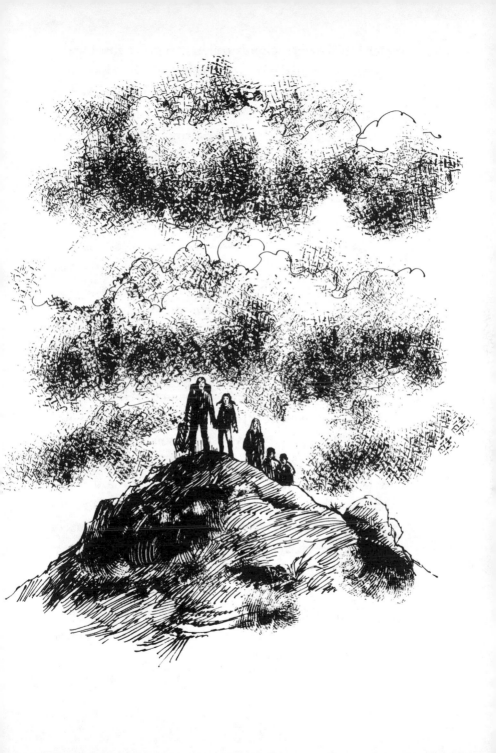

charcoal-colored clouds roiled across the just barely lighter gray of the evening sky.

Unmindful of the drizzle which streaked across their smudged faces, the five of them looked down the hillside to see a single brownish-gray thread strung through the darkness far below them.

"It's the road," Alana said hoarsely, still finding it hard to believe that they had indeed returned to the more familiar world outside of Pompey's Cave.

"What time is it, anyway?" Andy asked.

Without thinking, Chad moved his left wrist into the beam of the lantern. "Almost nine."

Alana gasped. "We were down there nearly twelve hours! It seemed like a . . ."

"Hey!" Sue interrupted indignantly. "Chad, when we were down in the cave, you said your watch wasn't working 'cause it got wet!"

The sandy-haired boy just looked at her helplessly. But Andy knew the reason Chad had not revealed the time before, and he tried to cover the awkward moment by saying, "Never mind about the watch—it's waterproof, I guess. I'm more interested in the Edison saying Chad must surely have for such an occasion."

Chad grinned at the good-natured teasing. "You know," he admitted, "I can't think of a thing!"

"Impossible!" Roy joined in, laughing. "When I get home, I'll have to read up on Edison just to find a quotation for you."

140

"Speaking of home," Sue reminded them. "Let's get going. I'm starving."

"You're always hungry," Andy said.

"No, I'm not."

"Yes, you are!"

"Oh, boy!" Roy groaned. "They're at it again. Come on, you two. We've still got a long walk home."

The trackless underbrush tore at their wet clothes as they carefully made their way down the hill toward the road. Only once did they pause when they had to cross a narrow rivulet of rainwater rushing down the side of the hill to the ancient creekbed below them to their left.

All five gazed down at the rocky channel they had walked on this morning. Dimly visible against the darker, leaf-covered creekbed were the upthrusting rocks that marked the entrance to Pompey's Cave.

"It seems like a lifetime ago," Alana murmured, putting into words what they all felt.

Then they resumed their trek down the hill, with Sue saying, "I never realized it could be so light at this time of night."

"Anywhere would be brighter than that cave," Andy told her.

But the scientist in Chad had been reawakened by Sue's question, and he explained as they went along, "The woods are never really pitch-dark even in the middle of the night. You just don't realize it until you're away from man-made illumination. It'll be darker when we get down off the hill, but it won't be too bad. We've still got the flashlights."

"*A* flashlight," Alana corrected, then waved her beamless flashlight when they looked around at her. "It just conked out," she told them. "Chad, you think the battery lantern will hold out till we get to a lighted road?"

Chad nodded. "The highway's less than a mile from here. Maybe we can hitch a ride into town from there."

"I hope so," Andy sighed. "But I'll be thankful just to feel level ground under me again."

A few minutes later, they were trudging down the dirt road that cleaved through the wilderness area of High Falls Park.

They had gone less than two hundred yards along this muddy track when the headlights of an approaching car knifed through the drizzle.

"I'll try to flag it down," Chad said, waving the lantern. "But I doubt if anyone will stop in such a desolate spot."

Chad was wrong, however.

As soon as the driver saw the weaving light, he applied his brakes, coming to a slithering, mud-splashing stop a few yards past them.

Alana suddenly gripped Chad's arm, words spilling from her lips in happy confusion.

"Oh, Chad! It's my parents! My mother and father have been looking for me!"

Then she was racing over the muddy road, her arms outstretched toward the man and woman who had just emerged from the waiting car.

17

Solving the Mysteries
of Pompey's Cave

Parents were a strange breed, the five explorers agreed when, a week later, they returned once more to Pompey's Cave. At first it had been "that horrible hole" and "that death trap," yet today those same parents had wholeheartedly agreed to let their children go back to the scene of their ordeal. Of course, the difference was that Professor O'Malley was going with them.

As an archaeologist, Alana's father had been immediately intrigued by the fossils Chad had persisted in carrying through Pompey's Cave. But it was the whole story of this "filling cave" which had caused the professor to spend almost a week digging through old records and journals at the state library as well as various historical societies.

Now, today, they were back in the dry creek-bed where their adventure had first started. After the "gully-washer" of a week ago, the leaves which covered the rocky bed were a plastered-down mass of brown pulp, and the sunlight glinted off the many shallow pools still remaining along the sides. The water there was unmoving, as if patiently waiting until it would be allowed to drain through one of the numerous leaf-stuffed cracks leading into the vast natural reservoir of which Pompey's Cave was only a part.

Professor O'Malley had promised the other parents that by no means would he permit their children to re-enter the cave, nor could they have done so at this point even if they had wanted to. For when they reached the shelving rocks where Roy's ladder had once led down into the shaft, they could hear the slosh of water even before they saw it.

Looking down into the shaft, a chill seemed to upthrust each and every hair on their bodies. Their signal pole was gone, its splinted body having been broken again by the surging flood. Nor was there any sign of it, except for a torn piece of yellow material—all that remained of Alana's scarf—caught in a piece of floating wood. Then as they watched, it, too, disappeared beneath the angry brown water that churned against the sides of the shaft less than ten feet from the surface where they stood.

"You were right, Chad," Roy half whispered. "The water didn't rise all the way up the shaft."

Professor O'Malley's blue eyes—so much like those of his daughter—were scanning the parts of the shaft visible above the water. "I doubt if it ever comes right up to the top—at least not nowadays."

"It sure comes high enough, though," Sue observed dolefully.

Alana's father nodded. "I hope all of you remember that. You know, you broke practically every rule of responsible caving—going off without telling anyone, without enough equipment . . ."

He stopped abruptly when he saw their downcast, embarrassed expressions. Then in a gentler tone, he went on, "But we've gone over all that before, and I don't doubt you now know—even better than I do—how important it is to follow such rules."

A smile played at the corners of his mouth. "From a purely selfish standpoint, however, I'm very glad you did go exploring—for more reasons than one."

He was looking directly at Alana, who smiled happily at his words, though she offered no explanation to the others.

In fact, Alana had been acting mighty secretive,

Chad reflected, as they began climbing the hill to what had been their exit from Pompey's Cave.

He and Alana had dropped behind the others, for the sandy-haired boy was intrigued by her exuberant yet enigmatic manner. He was hoping she might say something about it when Sue looked behind at the lagging pair.

"Watch out, Roy! He's at it again," she warned impishly. "He's trying to steal your girl."

Sue had not reckoned with Professor O'Malley, however. And his next words effectively silenced her—at least in reference to Alana's choice of company.

"Nobody is stealing Alana," he said without any irritation, but firmly enough that everyone knew he meant business. "The reason being that my daughter, at thirteen, is too young to be going steady with anyone. Nor does she want to. Therefore, Alana is nobody's girl—except mine, in a different sort of way."

"Yes, sir," Sue squeaked, causing what could have been a tense moment to be ruptured by the laughter of the others.

As they continued to climb the hill above the creekbed, Chad and Alana were still a few yards behind the main group. Professor O'Malley's statement had made a deep impression on the boy, but not in the way Sue might have thought it would.

148

He was struggling to put his idea into words when Alana solved the problem.

"About what I said in the cave," she began. "About my parents. Well, it just wasn't so. I was wrong. That night—after the cave—I told them how I felt, just as you said I should, Chad."

"That helped you to see things a little differently, huh?" he asked, remembering his own talk with his father.

"And how! They even want me to go along with them on their summer digs. They always thought I didn't want to go—it's really roughing it, you know—and that I had no interest in their work."

Chad grinned. "I guess that's what's called the generation gap, but it looks like you've managed to bridge it."

"Bridge it? You mean cave it—me and Pompey's Cave, plus a little help from Chad Evans," Alana said solemnly, then looked up at Chad with shining eyes. "You know, they told me something I never knew before—the reason why they called me Alana. It's a Gaelic word for 'beloved little girl.' "

Chad nodded. "I can see why they chose it," he told her softly. For a moment his eyes revealed his own feelings, but then he remembered Professor O'Malley's words and so Chad did not voice those thoughts. Instead, he took Alana's hand, squeezing it briefly, then began pulling her up the hill to where the others were now waiting at the exit of Pompey's Cave.

"There's where your barrel probably went down," Professor O'Malley stated, after measuring the width of the opening.

"But would it fit?" Andy asked. "I mean, between the hole and that boulder in front of it?"

"Well, I won't know till I see the barrel," Professor O'Malley began, but Sue interrupted.

"You can't see it. Roy broke it when he was hunting for the treasure!"

The older man's eyebrows lifted quizzically. "You mean Bootleg Brody's wealth?"

When Roy nodded, Alana's father chuckled. "Well, I guess a lot of people searched for it, but I wouldn't waste too much time on it, Roy."

"Why? Nobody found it, did they?"

"No, Roy, nobody did, so far as I could find out. However, I did learn that shortly after Brody was shot, his widow moved to Florida. It seems she bought a palatial home there, complete with swimming pool, servants—the works."

His meaning was obvious, but Sue felt the need to demonstrate that she understood too. "You mean Mrs. Bootleg Brody must have found all his money."

150

Nodding, the professor said, "As for the size of that barrel, Sue, even though the wooden staves are smashed, I can still measure the iron rims to determine its size."

While Sue was trying to figure that out, he went over to shine his flashlight down into the chamber where they had found the spiders. "I'm going to go down just to look around," he told them.

"Watch out for Big Pompey!" Sue warned.

"Gosh, I thought you'd forgotten about that!" Andy chided.

Alana's father paused before ducking into the entrance to the upper chamber. "Big Pompey, the snake-lizard that guards Brody's treasure? I came across that interesting bit of folklore in my research. Certainly you don't believe it, do you, Sue?"

"Well . . . no . . . but . . ."

"If I was a bootlegger using the cave as a store-house," he explained patiently, "I'd try to find some way to keep people out, wouldn't you?"

"Oh, I see!" Sue exclaimed. "Brody made up the story so he could have the cave all to himself."

Professor O'Malley nodded. "That's one possibility. The story might also have been invented by parents who wanted to make sure that inquisitive youngsters wouldn't go stumbling around in there and get lost."

151

"Oh . . ." The single word came out as a small whisper.

Patting the girl's shoulder to show he had not really meant it as a personal rebuke, Professor O'Malley left the others sitting outside while he went down to examine the chamber.

They could see the beam of his flashlight flirting in and out among the rocks below, and once a short "Well, what do you know!" echoed up from the depths. Then all was silent for the next twenty minutes until the professor's smiling face appeared at the opening.

"Now I'm even more anxious to see the rest of the cave," he told them. "But I know I'll have to wait until the water recedes. Anyway, that chamber definitely has been used for human habitation."

"Did you see the pile of wood over near the entrance to the tunnel?" Roy asked.

The professor nodded enthusiastically. "That was a ladder all right—see." He was holding up a bent and rusted nail.

"What do you think about the cave being used as a stop on the Underground Railroad?" Chad wanted to know.

Professor O'Malley thought for a minute, then told them, "When I saw the entrance you first showed me," and he pointed down the hill toward the creekbed, "I'd have said that story was prob-

152

ably just folklore. After all, that section of the cave is sometimes under water and, aside from the danger it presents, it couldn't be depended on as a hideout."

Alana was leaning forward expectantly.

"However, after I've seen this upper chamber," her father continued, "I'd say it might well have been used to hide escaped slaves. Of course, there wouldn't be much about it in old records—there was a law against aiding fugitive slaves even up here in the North. But this nail is handmade, and certainly predates the time Brody used the cave."

"Predates?" Sue questioned.

"It's older than the 1920's," Andy impatiently explained.

"That's all I was waiting to hear," Alana spoke up. Bending over to rummage through the satchel she had been carrying, she lifted out a rusted object that resembled a saucer with a handle.

Turning to the quartet of young people, she said, "Remember when we were climbing out of there last Saturday and I lagged behind? Well, this is what I found." Then her eyes locked on those of her father as he reached forward to receive the rusted piece of iron.

"Unless I miss my guess, it . . . it's an old-fashioned candleholder!" he exclaimed. "Why didn't you . . ."

"I wasn't sure. I thought maybe it was just a

153

piece of junk and that you'd laugh or . . . well, you know," Alana concluded in confusion.

"Laugh? I'd never do that," her father assured her. "Why, girl, you've got a genuine archaeological eye. I don't think I'd ever have spotted something like that when I was your age!"

Alana flushed with pleasure. "Then you think this really might have been left there by some fugitive slave?"

"Well, I can't be certain of that. But it adds weight to the story about Pompey's Cave being a stop on the Underground Railroad. Many things point to it—the entrance to the upper chamber is well camouflaged by that boulder, and in the summer the underbrush would make it practically invisible. Then there's the ladder and the arrow . . ."

"What about the arrow?" Chad broke in. "Who do you think carved . . ." Then realizing he had interrupted Alana's father, he apologized and sat back to listen.

"That's alright, Chad. I can well understand your enthusiasm," Professor O'Malley told him. "As for the arrow, I doubt if there's any way we can determine who chiseled it into the rock. But I don't think it was recent, because I found absolutely no mention of the upper chamber or how it connects to the entrance in the creekbed. The author of Roy's article obviously didn't know about it either,

154

and thought the cave only extended from the west lake to the smaller lake at the end of the east tunnel. And so far as I can tell, there's been nothing published about the cave since that time."

"I'd like to think the man who discovered the cave scratched the arrow in there," Alana said. "Maybe so nobody would get lost—like that poor slave woman with her baby."

"You might just be right," Professor O'Malley nodded. "As I said before, it would have been this upper chamber that was used to hide the slaves —any other place in the cave would have been too dangerous. But at times it might have been necessary to use the creekbed entrance, and the arrow would point the way to the upper chamber. In addition, the other entrance would provide an escape route—at least in dry weather—if someone found the opening here."

"Fossils, treasure, escaped slaves, a snake-lizard, and a bootlegger—whew!" Andy summed it all up.

"Oh, yes, fossils!" Professor O'Malley exclaimed. "One of those you showed me was definitely a Murchisonia—probably from the Silurian Period, which occurred between 405 and 425 million years ago."

"Wow!"

"Make that a double wow, Sue," he instructed.

155

"Although Silurian outcroppings are common in eastern North America, I've never known of any found in this immediate area. That's why I intend to lead an exploration team down there as soon as it's possible."

Professor O'Malley paused a moment, then added, "Of course, we'll need a guide . . ."

"Not me!" Sue and Andy chorused, for once in perfect harmony of thought.

"And I've got two left feet when it comes to direction," Alana assured them.

Draping his arm around Chad's shoulder, Roy looked at the boy he had once derisively called "Bumblefoot."

Seeing the question in Roy's eyes, Chad nodded, knowing the dark-haired athlete would have no qualms about going back down into the cave. In any event, Roy's parents would surely give their permission since he would be guiding a group of scientists, some of whom were experienced spelunkers.

Yet, surprisingly, Roy did not choose the limelight for himself, as he so often had done on the football field. Instead, he told Professor O'Malley, "With his scientific mind and all, Chad is the best guide you could find."

Grinning broadly after the first moment of

156

stunned silence, Chad was quick to interject, "Only when I'm with my partner, Roy."

As the others watched, the two friends solemnly shook hands. Then the group started back down the hill, satisfied that some of the mysteries had been solved, but looking forward to others that might still be hidden deep within Pompey's Cave.

About the Author

PATRICIA EDWARDS CLYNE was born in New York City and graduated with a BA degree in journalism from Hunter College. She worked as a reporter and also as a free-lance editor.

Early childhood visits to Ozark Mountain caves resulted in a lifelong interest which is now centered on rock shelters of the Northeast, many of which she has investigated and photographed for her articles and stories. Her new novel, *Tunnels of Terror*, is set in one of the caves of the Northeast, which she has explored along with her family.

Mrs. Clyne lives in New York with her husband and four sons, all of whom share in her love of exploring and hiking. She is the author of one previous juvenile book, *The Corduroy Road*.

About the Artist

FRANK ALOISE studied at the Art Students League, The Workshop School of Art, and the School of Visual Arts in New York. He worked in the graphics department of NBC for several years before going into free-lance book illustrating.

Mr. Aloise has received merit awards from the Art Directors Club of New York and the Society of Illustrators, and has had exhibitions of his oils, water colors, and etchings.

He lives with his wife, Priscilla, and their daughter, Kate, in New York City.